FATTY-LIVER COOKBOOK

Revive Your Liver with Flavorful Recipes: A Guide to Healthy Eating for Fatty Liver.

Roslin Shelton

Thank you for choosing my book and recipes. I have worked hard for it, your positive review on Amazon would help me a lot.

Greetings Roslin Shelton.

DOWNLOAD YOUR BONUS

Table of Contents

Introduction

Steatosis Hepatica, also known as Fatty Liver Disease, is a condition in which excessive fat accumulates in the liver. This can happen in individuals who consume too much alcohol or who have a poor diet and sedentary lifestyle, but it can also affect non-drinkers and those who are otherwise healthy.

The condition occurs when the liver cannot break down fats efficiently, leading to an accumulation of fat in the liver cells. Over time, this can cause inflammation and scarring in the liver, which can further damage its function. If left untreated, it can progress to more serious conditions, such as cirrhosis of the liver.

Common symptoms of Fatty Liver Disease include fatigue, abdominal pain, and swelling in the legs or abdomen. However, many people may experience no symptoms at all, making it important to get regular check-ups with a doctor to monitor liver health.

Fortunately, Fatty Liver Disease can often be managed or even reversed through lifestyle changes such as a healthy diet, regular exercise, and moderate alcohol consumption or abstinence. If you are concerned about your liver health, speak to your doctor about getting tested for Fatty Liver Disease and how you can take steps to improve your liver health.

Fatty liver disease is a condition that affects many people worldwide. It occurs when too much fat accumulates in the liver, which can lead to various complications such as liver failure, cirrhosis, and even liver cancer. For those living with fatty liver disease, making dietary changes is crucial to manage symptoms and improve liver function.

This recipe book is designed to provide healthy eating options for people with fatty liver disease. We have carefully selected ingredients that are nutritious and beneficial for your liver, such as lean proteins, high-fiber grains, fruits, vegetables, and healthy fats. Our recipes are easy to prepare, affordable, and satisfying, suitable for a range of occasions, from a quick breakfast to a hearty dinner.

It's important to note that while making dietary changes can be beneficial, it's nonetheless essential to work with a healthcare professional to manage your fatty liver disease. This recipe book should not replace any medical advice and is intended to be used in conjunction with your healthcare provider's recommendations.

Overall, our objective is to inspire people with fatty liver disease to cook delicious, healthy meals that can help manage their condition and optimize their overall health.

Brief description of fatty liver disease

Fatty liver disease or hepatic steatosis is a condition characterized by the accumulation of fat in the liver cells. This is usually caused by excessive alcohol consumption, obesity, or diabetes. As the liver is responsible for a variety of crucial functions such as filtering toxic substances out of the blood, producing bile, and regulating glucose levels in the blood, the buildup of fat in its cells can lead to inflammation, scarring, and liver damage over time. Fatty liver disease is often asymptomatic, but in some cases, it can cause fatigue, abdominal discomfort, and jaundice. To treat the condition, it is important to address the underlying causes such as losing weight, limiting alcohol consumption, and managing blood sugar levels for diabetic patients.

Symptoms of fatty liver disease

Fatty liver disease, or steatosis hepatica, may not always cause noticeable symptoms. However, when symptoms do occur, they can include:

- Fatigue and weakness

- Weight loss or unintended weight gain

- Abdominal pain and swelling

- Loss of appetite

- Nausea and vomiting

- Jaundice (yellowing of the skin and eyes)

- Confusion or difficulty concentrating

- Spider-like blood vessels on the skin

- Red palms

It's important to note that Fatty Liver Disease can progress to more severe conditions, such as liver fibrosis and cirrhosis, which can cause additional symptoms like easy bruising, itching, and swelling in the legs and ankles.

If you are experiencing any of the symptoms listed above or have concerns about your liver health, it's important to speak with your doctor as soon as possible. They can help you determine the underlying cause of your symptoms and develop a treatment plan to manage the condition.

Diagnosis of Fatty Liver Disease (Steatosis Hepatica)

Fatty liver disease, or steatosis hepatica, can be diagnosed through a variety of tests and imaging procedures. These may include:

1. Blood tests: A blood test can reveal elevated levels of liver enzymes, which indicate that the liver is inflamed and not functioning properly.

2. Imaging tests: Imaging tests such as ultrasound, CT scans, or magnetic resonance imaging (MRI) can be used to detect excess fat in the liver.

3. Biopsy: In some cases, a liver biopsy may be necessary to confirm the diagnosis. During a biopsy, a small sample of liver tissue is removed and examined in a lab for signs of fatty liver disease.

It's important to note that fatty liver disease can sometimes be confused with other liver conditions or diseases. Therefore, it's important to see a doctor who can conduct the appropriate tests and make an accurate diagnosis.

General Dietary Recommendations for People with Fatty Liver Disease (Steatosis Hepatica)

Adopting a healthy diet is an important part of managing fatty liver disease. Below are some general dietary guidelines that can help:

1. Reduce your intake of saturated and trans fats: These types of fats are found in high amounts in fried foods, fatty meats, and processed snacks. They can contribute to the buildup of fat in the liver. Instead, focus on consuming monounsaturated and polyunsaturated fats such as those found in nuts, seeds, avocado, and fatty fish like salmon.

2. Reduce your intake of sugar and refined carbohydrates: These include foods such as candy, cookies, white bread, and sugary drinks. They can contribute to insulin resistance, which can worsen fatty liver disease. Instead, choose whole grains, fruits, and vegetables as your main sources of carbohydrates.

3. Increase your intake of fiber: Fiber helps to promote digestion and can help to improve insulin sensitivity. Excellent sources of fiber include fruits, legumes, nuts, whole grains, and vegetables.

4. Limit alcohol intake: Alcohol consumption can increase the risk of liver damage and should be avoided or consumed in moderation. Experts recommend no more than one or two drinks a day for both women and men.

5. Drink plenty of water: Staying hydrated is important for overall health and can help support liver function.

It's important to note that dietary recommendations may vary depending on the severity of the fatty liver disease and other health conditions. Therefore, it's always best to consult with a registered dietitian or healthcare provider for personalized nutrition advice.

Foods not recommended for fatty liver disease

1. Saturated fats: Found in high-fat dairy products, fatty meats, and tropical oils such as coconut and palm oil. Consuming too much saturated fat can contribute to the buildup of fat in the liver, making fatty liver disease worse.

2. Trans fats: These are found in many processed foods, including fried foods, baked goods, and snack foods. Trans fats can raise levels of LDL (bad) cholesterol and contribute to insulin resistance, both of which can exacerbate fatty liver disease.

3. Added sugars: These include the sugars added to processed foods, desserts, and sugary drinks. Excess sugar consumption can contribute to the development of insulin resistance and increase the risk of fatty liver disease.

4. Refined carbohydrates: These include white bread, white rice, and other processed grain products. They can contribute to insulin resistance and inflammation, which can worsen fatty liver disease.

5. Alcohol: Drinking alcohol can put additional strain on the liver, making fatty liver disease worse. Experts recommend that those with fatty liver disease eliminate or significantly reduce their alcohol intake.

It's important to note that everyone's dietary needs and restrictions can vary based on their individual health conditions and other factors. Therefore, it's recommended to consult with a healthcare provider or a registered dietitian before making major dietary changes or eliminating any major food groups.

Foods recommended for fatty liver

There are several healthy ingredients that are recommended for individuals with fatty liver disease (steatosis hepatica). Here are some examples:

1. Fiber-rich foods: Include fruits, vegetables, whole grains, and legumes in your diet. These foods can help with weight loss and improve insulin sensitivity, which can help reduce the buildup of fat in the liver.

2. Lean protein: Choose lean sources of protein such as fish, chicken, turkey, legumes, and tofu. These foods provide important nutrients while being low in saturated fat.

3. Healthy fats: Unprocessed plant-based oils such as olive oil, avocado oil, and canola oil, nuts and seeds like almonds, chia, flaxseeds, and walnuts are good options for healthy fats that can help improve liver function

4. Low glycemic index foods: These are foods that do not cause a large spike in blood glucose levels. Examples include sweet potatoes, whole grains, and most fruits.

5. Water: Drinking plenty of water can help flush toxins from the body and keep the liver functioning properly.

It is important to note that dietary restrictions and nutritional needs may vary based on an individual's health condition and other factors. Therefore, it's recommended to consult with a healthcare provider or a registered dietitian before making major dietary changes or eliminating any major food groups.

Behavioral advice for those suffering from fatty liver disease

1. Maintain a healthy weight: Being overweight or obese can increase the risk of fatty liver disease. Losing weight and maintaining a healthy weight can reduce fat accumulation in the liver and improve liver function.

2. Exercise regularly: Regular exercise can help with weight loss and improve insulin sensitivity, which can help reduce fat deposition in the liver. Low-impact exercises such as walking, cycling, or swimming can be beneficial.

3. Avoid alcohol: Alcohol can cause inflammation and damage to the liver, which can worsen fatty liver disease. Individuals with fatty liver disease should avoid or limit alcohol intake.

4. Quit smoking: Smoking can also contribute to liver damage and worsen fatty liver disease. Quitting smoking can improve liver function and overall health.

5. Eat a well-balanced diet: Opt for a nutritious diet that avoids excessive saturated fats, added sugars, and processed foods as this could be beneficial for people diagnosed with hepatic steatosis. Consuming a variety of whole grains, fruits, vegetables, and lean protein sources can potentially aid in improving liver health.

6. Control other pre-existing health conditions: It is possible that people with fatty liver disease may have other illnesses such as type 2 diabetes, high blood pressure, and high cholesterol. Successfully managing these medical conditions through medications or lifestyle changes, or a combination of both, could also enhance liver function.

It's important to note that these tips are general recommendations and may need to be modified depending on an individual's health status and needs. Therefore, it's recommended to consult with a healthcare provider or a registered dietitian to develop a personalized plan for managing fatty liver disease.

Recommendation and advice

Before beginning any type of diet, it is important to consult with a healthcare provider or registered dietitian. They can help determine if the diet is appropriate for individual needs and health conditions, as well as providing guidance on how to safely achieve any desired goals.

It is also important to note that diets that promise rapid weight loss may not be sustainable or healthy in the long term. It's important to focus on making dietary changes that can be maintained over time to achieve lasting health benefits.

In addition, individuals with certain health conditions, such as diabetes or kidney disease, may need to modify certain aspects of their diet to manage their condition effectively.

Overall, seeking the guidance and support of a healthcare professional can help ensure that any dietary changes are safe, effective, and sustainable in the long term.

Breakfast

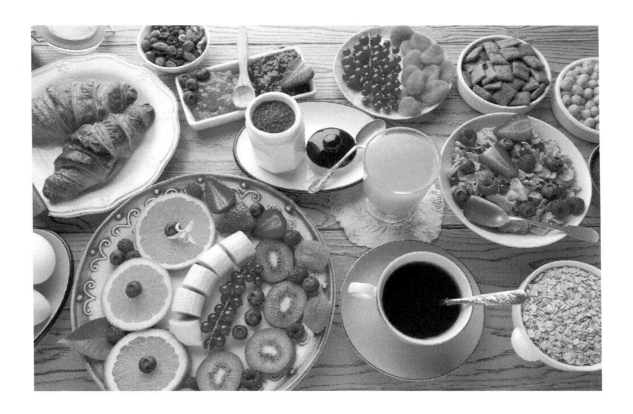

1. Low-carb Scrambled Eggs

- Difficulty: Easy   Preparation Time: 6 minutes
- Cooking Time: 6 minutes   Serving: 1
- Ingredients:
- 2 large eggs
- 1 tbsp. unsweetened almond milk
- 1/4 cup chopped spinach
- 1 tsp olive oil
- Salt and pepper

Instructions:

1. In a bowl, whisk together the almond milk and eggs until blended.
2. Heat the oil over medium heat in a nonstick skillet.
3. Place the chopped spinach in the pan and sauté 1 minute, until wilted.
4. Add the egg mixture to the pan and mix gently with a paddle.
5. Cook for 3-4 minutes, stirring occasionally, until the eggs are fully cooked.
6. Season with salt and pepper.
7. Serve and enjoy your meal.

Nutritional Values per Person:

Calories: 185 Protein: 14g Carbohydrates: 2g Fat: 13g Fiber: 1g

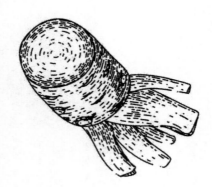

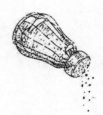

2. Quinoa Breakfast Bowl

Difficulty: Easy   Preparation Time: 12 minutes

Cooking Time: 22 minutes Serving: 2

Ingredients:

- 1/2 cup quinoa
- 1 cup water
- 2 tbsp. olive oil
- 1 medium sweet potato, peeled and cubed
- 1/4 tsp garlic powder
- 1/4 tsp paprika
- 1/4 tsp salt
- 2 cups baby spinach
- 4 large eggs
- Salt and pepper

Instructions:

1. Rinse the quinoa and add it to a pot with water. Turn it on and bring it to a boil, then turn the heat down to low and simmer for 15 minutes or until the quinoa absorbs the water.
2. Turn the heat up in another pan and heat the olive oil over medium heat.
3. Add the sweet potato cubes and stir to coat. Sprinkle with garlic powder, paprika and salt, then let it cook for about 10 minutes or until soft and golden brown.
4. Add baby spinach to the pan and cook until wilted.
5. Fry the eggs in a non-stick pan until desired consistency.
6. Divide cooked quinoa into two bowls, then divide sweet potato and spinach mixture equally.
7. Top each bowl with 2 fried eggs and season with salt and pepper.

Nutritional Values per Person:

- Calories: 395
- Protein: 17g
- Carbohydrates: 29g
- Fat: 23g
- Fiber: 5g

3. Coconut Flour Pancakes

Difficulty: Easy   Preparation Time: 10 minutes

Cooking Time: 10 minutes Serving: 2-3

Ingredients:

- 1/2 cup coconut flour
- 1/2 tsp baking powder
- 1/4 tsp salt
- 4 large eggs
- 1/3 cup unsweetened almond milk
- 1/4 cup coconut oil
- 1 tsp vanilla extract
- Optional: fresh berries for topping

Instructions:

1. 1.In a bowl, mix the coconut flour, baking powder, and salt.
2. In another mixing bowl, beat the eggs until light and frothy.
3. Add almond milk, melted coconut oil and vanilla extract into the beaten eggs, and mix well.
4. Add dry ingredients into wet ingredients, and mix until fully combined.
5. Place a non-stick pan on medium heat.
6. Using a quarter cup measuring cup, pour the batter onto the skillet.
7. Cook the pancake until the edges start to brown and the surface is bubbly, then flip and cook for another minute or until golden brown.
8. Repeat with the remaining batter.

Nutritional Values per Person: Calories: 325 Protein: 12g Carbohydrates: 14g Fat: 26g Fiber: 8g

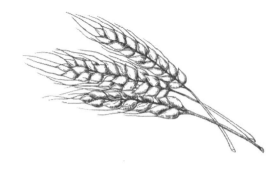

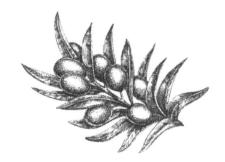

4. Gypsy Toast

Difficulty: Easy   Preparation Time: 10 minutes

Cooking Time: 17 minutes Serving: 2

Ingredients:

- 1 head of broccoli, cut into small florets
- 2 tbsp. olive oil
- 1/4 cup whole wheat flour
- 1/4 cup grated Parmesan cheese
- 1/4 tsp garlic powder
- Salt and pepper to taste
- 1 egg, lightly beaten
- Cooking spray

Instructions:

1. Turn on the oven and bring it to 375°F (190°C).
2. In a mixing bowl, combine the flour, Parmesan cheese, salt, pepper and garlic powder.
3. Add the broccoli florets to the bowl and mix until the florets are coated in the flour mixture.
4. Dip each broccoli floret into the beaten egg mixture, shaking off any excess.
5. Arrange the coated broccoli florets on a baking tray with parchment paper.
6. Lightly spray the broccoli florets with cooking spray.
7. Bake the broccoli poppers in the preheated oven for 22-27 minutes until crisp and golden brown.
8. Once done, take the pan out of the oven and let it rest for 6-7 minutes.
9. Transfer the roasted broccoli poppers to a serving bowl and serve as a healthy snack.

Nutritional Values per Serving: Calories: 130 Fat: 8g Carbohydrates: 11g Fiber: 4g Protein: 6g

5. Dreamy Vanilla Chia Seed Pudding

Difficulty: Easy   **Preparation Time: 10 minutes**

Cooking Time: 0 minutes   **Serving: 2**

Ingredients:

- 1/4 cup chia seeds
- 1 cup unsweetened almond milk
- 1/4 tsp vanilla extract
- 1 tbsp maple syrup
- Optional toppings: fresh berries, nuts, cinnamon

Instructions:

1. In a bowl, whisk together chia seeds, almond milk, vanilla extract and maple syrup.
2. Whisk until well combined and there are no clumps of chia seeds.
3. Cover and refrigerate for at least 3 hours or until the next day.
4. Before serving, give the pudding a good stir to ensure it's evenly mixed.
5. Serve chilled with your desired toppings.

Nutritional Values per Person: Calories: 120 Protein: 4g Carbohydrates: 12g Fat: 7g Fiber: 10g

6. Sweet Potato Hash with Sausage and Eggs

Difficulty: Easy   **Preparation Time: 10 minutes**

Cooking Time: 27 minutes   **Serving: 2**

Ingredients:

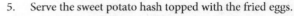

- 2 diced medium sized sweet potatoes
- 2 chicken sausages, sliced
- 1/2 diced onion
- 1 diced red pepper
- 1/4 tsp garlic powder
- 1/2 tsp smoked paprika
- Salt and pepper
- 2 tbsp olive oil
- 2 eggs

Instructions:

1. Turn on the medium-high heat and heat the oil in a large frying pan.
2. Add sweet potatoes and cook for about 8-10 minutes until they start to brown.
3. Add chicken sausages, onion, bell pepper, garlic powder, smoked paprika, pepper and salt, and cook for another 8-10 minutes until the vegetables are tender and the sausages are browned.
4. In a separate skillet, fry two eggs to your desired level of doneness.

5. Serve the sweet potato hash topped with the fried eggs.

Nutritional Values per Person: Calories: 450 Protein: 22g Carbohydrates: 30g Fat: 28g Fiber: 6g

7. Sweet Potato Toast with Avocado and Egg

Difficulty: Easy   **Preparation Time: 5 minutes**

Cooking Time: 20 minutes   **Serving: 2**

Ingredients:

- 1 large sweet potato, sliced into 1/4 inch thick pieces
- 1 ripe avocado
- 2 eggs
- Salt and pepper
- 1 tbsp. olive oil

Instructions:

1. Turn the oven on and bring it to 400°F.
2. Place a parchment paper on top of the baking sheet.
3. Cut the sweet potato into 1/4-inch thick pieces and arrange them on the baking sheet.
4. Brush each slice with olive oil and sprinkle with pepper and salt.
5. Cook for 15-20 minutes, turning the slices halfway through cooking, until lightly crisp and tender.
6. While the sweet potato toasts are baking, prepare the avocado and eggs.
7. In a small bowl, mash the avocado with a fork.
8. In a separate skillet, fry two eggs to your desired level of doneness.
9. Once the sweet potato toasts are done, remove from the oven and spread a layer of mashed avocado on each slice.
10. Cover each slice with a fried egg and sprinkle with pepper and salt.

Nutritional Values per Person: Calories: 340 Protein: 12g Carbohydrates: 25g Fat: 24g Fiber: 8g

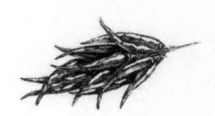

8. Healthy Smoked Salmon Breakfast Bagel

Difficulty: Easy   Preparation Time: 10 minutes

Cooking Time: 10 minutes Serving: 2 persons

Ingredients:

- 2 whole-wheat bagels
- 4 oz. smoked salmon
- 2 tbsp. light cream cheese
- 2 leaves of lettuce
- 2 slices of tomato
- 1/4 red onion, thinly sliced
- 1 tbsp. capers
- Salt and pepper

Instructions:

1. Turn the oven to 350°F (175°C) and prepare a baking sheet.
2. Cut the whole-wheat bagels in half and place them onto the prepared baking sheet.
3. Spread the light cream cheese on each half of the bagel and sprinkle with salt and pepper.
4. Bake the bagels for 10 to 12 minutes or until lightly browned and toasted.
5. While the bagels are baking, prepare the other ingredients. Wash the lettuce leaves and slice the tomato and red onion.
6. Once the bagels are done baking, remove them from the oven and place a lettuce leaf, two slices of smoked salmon, tomato, red onion, and capers on top of each half of the bagel.
7. Season with additional salt and pepper if desired or sprinkle with fresh herbs.
8. Top with the remaining half of the bagel and serve immediately.

Nutritional Values per Person: Calories: 293.2 Fat: 7.6g Carbohydrates: 35.9g Fiber: 6.8g Protein: 21.4g

9. Omelette with Spinach and Mushrooms

Difficulty: Easy   Preparation Time: 10 minutes

Cooking Time: 10 minutes Serving: 1

Ingredients:

- 3 large eggs
- ½ cup baby spinach, chopped
- ½ cup mushrooms, sliced
- 1 tbsp. olive oil
- Salt and pepper

Instructions:

1. Crack the eggs into a mixing bowl and whisk them together until they're completely combined. Set aside.
2. Turn the heat up and heat a nonstick skillet over medium heat with 1 tablespoon of the olive oil.
3. Add the mushrooms to the skillet and sauté for 2-3 minutes, or until they start to brown.
4. Add the spinach to the skillet and cook until wilted, about 1 to 2 minutes.
5. Pour the beaten eggs over the spinach and mushrooms, and use a spatula to evenly distribute the vegetables.
6. Cook until the edges of the omelette start to turn golden brown and the center is almost set.
7. Use a spatula to fold the omelette in half and slide it onto a plate.
8. Season with salt and pepper and serve immediately.

Nutritional Values per Person: Calories: 290 Protein: 21g Carbohydrates: 4g Fat: 22g Fiber: 1g

10. Green Smoothie Bowl

Difficulty: Easy   Preparation Time: 10 minutes

Cooking Time: 0 minutes   Serving: 1

Ingredients:

- 1 banana, frozen
- ½ avocado, pitted
- 1 cup baby spinach
- ½ cup unsweetened almond milk
- 1 tbsp. honey
- 1 tbsp. chia seeds
- 2 tbsp.
- Rolled oats
- ½ cup ice cubes

Instructions:

1. Place all ingredients in a blender and blend until smooth and creamy.
2. Pour the smoothie into a bowl.
3. Add toppings like fresh fruit, nuts, seeds, or granola.

Nutritional Values per Person: Calories: 440 Protein: 9g Carbohydrates: 59g Fat: 23g Fiber: 13g

11. Cottage Cheese and Peach Salad

Difficulty: Easy   Preparation Time: 12 minutes

Cooking Time: 0 minutes   Serving: 2

Ingredients:

- 1 cup of cottage cheese
- 2 peaches, sliced
- 2 cups of mixed greens (such as spinach or arugula)
- 1/4 cup of chopped walnuts
- 1 tbsp. of balsamic vinegar
- 1 tbsp. of olive oil
- Salt and pepper

Instructions:

1. In a large bowl, combine the cottage cheese, sliced peaches, and mixed greens.
2. In a bowl, whisk together the olive oil and balsamic vinegar.
3. Combine the dressing over the salad and mix.
4. Season with salt and pepper.
5. Divide the salad between two bowls.
6. Sprinkle with chopped walnuts.
7. Serve and enjoy!

Nutritional Values per Person: Calories: 275 Protein: 18g Carbohydrates: 25g Fat: 12g Fiber: 5g

12. Tuna and Vegetable Frittata

Difficulty: Easy   Preparation Time: 12 minutes

Cooking Time: 15 minutes Serving: 4

Ingredients:

- 4 eggs
- 1 can of tuna in water, drained and flaked
- 1 cup of mixed vegetables, chopped (such as bell peppers, onions, and mushrooms)
- ½ cup of grated low-fat cheese
- 1 tbsp. of olive oil
- Salt and pepper to taste

Instructions:

1. Turn on the oven and bring it to 350°F (175°C).
2. Season the eggs in a bowl with salt and pepper to taste and beat them.
3. Turn on the medium heat and heat a pan with the oil.
4. Add the mixed vegetables to the skillet and sauté for 5 minutes or until tender.
5. Add the flaked tuna to the vegetables and stir together.
6. Pour the beaten eggs over the vegetables and tuna in the skillet.

7. Sprinkle the grated cheese on top.
8. Cook the eggs in the oven until the cheese has melted and the eggs are solidified
9. Remove the skillet from the oven and let it cool.
10. Slice the frittata into 4 portions.
11. Serve hot and enjoy!

Nutritional Values per Person: Calories: 180 Protein: 18g Carbohydrates: 3g Fat: 11g Fiber: 1g

13. Cozy Apple Cinnamon Oatmeal

Difficulty: Easy   Preparation Time: 5 minutes

Cooking Time: 12 minutes Serving: 2

Ingredients:

- 1 cup of rolled oats
- 2 cups of water
- 1 apple, diced
- 1 tsp of cinnamon
- 1 tbsp. of honey
- 2 tbsp. of chopped nuts (such as almonds or walnuts

Instructions:

1. In a saucepan, bring the water to a boil.
2. Add the rolled oats to the boiling water and stir.
3. Reduce the heat to low and cook for 5 to 7 minutes, stirring occasionally, until the oats are soft and creamy.
4. Add the diced apple, cinnamon, and honey to the oatmeal and stir until combined.
5. Divide the oatmeal between two bowls.
6. Garnish each bowl with chopped nuts.
7. Serve hot and enjoy!

Nutritional Values per Person: Calories: 250 Protein: 6g Carbohydrates: 45g Fat: 6g Fiber: 7g

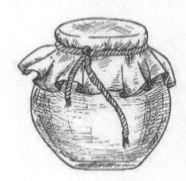

14. Avocado Toast with Smoked Salmon

Difficulty: Easy   Preparation Time: 10 minutes

Cooking Time: 0 minutes   Serving: 2

Ingredients:

- 2 slices of whole-grain bread
- 1 ripe avocado
- 1 lemon
- Salt and pepper
- 2 oz. smoked salmon
- Fresh dill

Instructions:

1. Toast the bread until lightly browned.
2. While the bread toasts, cut the avocado, remove the pit and place the pulp in a small bowl. With a fork, mash the pulp and add a squeeze of lemon juice. Mix well.
3. Season the avocado mixture with salt and pepper.
4. Lay a slice of smoked salmon on each piece of toast.
5. Spread the mashed avocado mixture generously on top of the smoked salmon.
6. Garnish with fresh dill.
7. Serve and enjoy!

Nutritional Values per Person: Calories: 310 Protein: 13g Carbohydrates: 30g Fat: 16g Fiber: 10g

15. Smoothie with Beetroot and Carrot

Difficulty: Easy   Preparation Time: 12 minutes

Cooking Time: 0 minutes   Serving: 2

Ingredients:

- 1 medium beetroot, peeled and chopped
- 1 medium carrot, peeled and chopped
- 1 banana
- 1 cup of almond milk
- 1 tbsp. of honey
- 1 tsp of ground ginger
- 1 cup of ice

Instructions:

1. Add the chopped beetroot and carrot to a blender.
2. Peel and slice the banana, then add it to the blender.
3. Pour in the almond milk, honey, ground ginger, and ice.
4. Blend until smooth and creamy.
5. Check the consistency and adjust it by adding more ice or milk if necessary.
6. Divide the smoothie into two glasses.
7. Serve and enjoy!

Nutritional Values per Person: Calories: 168 Protein: 3.5g Carbohydrates: 33.5g Fat: 3.5g Fiber: 8g

16. Spinach and Mushroom Omelet

Difficulty: Easy   Preparation Time: 12 minutes

Cooking Time: 12 minutes Serving: 1

Ingredients:

- 2 large eggs
- 1/2 cup of spinach, washed and chopped
- 1/4 cup of mushrooms, sliced
- 1 tbsp. of olive oil
- Salt and pepper

Instructions:

1. Place the eggs in a small bowl and beat them with a fork.
2. Turn the heat to medium and heat the oil in a non-stick pan.
3. Add sliced mushrooms and sauté for 2-3 minutes until browned, stirring occasionally.
4. Add spinach to the skillet and sauté for an additional 2-3 minutes until wilted.
5. Pour the eggs into the pan and cook for 2-3 minutes, or until the underside is cooked through.
6. Fold the omelet in half with a spatula and cook another minute or until the eggs are fully cooked.
7. Season with salt and pepper.
8. Serve and enjoy your Mushroom and Spinach Omelet!

Nutritional Values per Person: Calories: 225 Protein: 14g Carbohydrates: 3g Fat: 17g Fiber: 1g

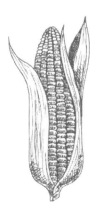

17. Mixed Berry Smoothie

Difficulty: Easy   Preparation Time: 6 minutes

Cooking Time: 0 minutes   Serving: 1

Ingredients:

- 1/2 cup mixed berries (fresh or frozen)
- 1/2 cup unsweetened almond milk
- 1/2 cup plain Greek yogurt
- 1 tsp honey
- 1/2 tsp vanilla extract
- Ice cubes (optional)

Instructions:

1. Add the mixed berries, unsweetened almond milk, Greek yogurt, honey, and vanilla extract to a blender.
2. If desired, add ice cubes to the blender to create a thicker consistency.
3. Blend all ingredients until smooth and creamy.
4. Taste and adjust sweetness with additional honey, if necessary.
5. Pour the smoothie into a glass and serve immediately.

Nutritional Values per Person: Calories: 205 Protein: 19g Carbohydrates: 24g Fat: 5g Fiber: 4g

18. Chia Seed Pudding with Berries

Difficulty: Easy   Preparation Time: 10 minutes (plus 2-3 hours of chilling time)

Cooking Time: 0 minutes   Serving: 2

Ingredients:

- 1/4 cup chia seeds
- 1 cup unsweetened almond milk
- 1 tbsp. honey
- 1/2 tsp vanilla extract
- 1/2 cup mixed berries (fresh or frozen)
- 2 tbsp. sliced almonds (optional)

Instructions:

1. In a bowl, add the chia seeds, honey, vanilla extract and unsweetened almond milk.
2. Whisk the mixture well for a few minutes until the chia seeds are evenly distributed.
3. Cover the bowl and place it in the refrigerator for at least 2-3 hours or until the next day.
4. Once the chia pudding has chilled and thickened, spoon it into two separate serving dishes.
5. Top each serving with a handful of mixed berries and sliced almonds, if desired.
6. Serve and enjoy!

Nutritional Values per Person: Calories: 200 Protein: 6g Carbohydrates: 22g Fat: 9g Fiber: 14g

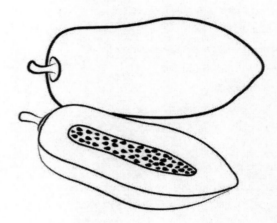

19. Peanut Butter Banana Smoothie

Difficulty: Easy   Preparation Time: 5 minutes

Cooking Time: 0 minutes   Serving: 2

Ingredients:

- 2 ripe bananas
- 2 tbsp. peanut butter
- 1 cup unsweetened almond milk
- 1 tbsp. honey
- 1/2 tsp vanilla extract
- 1 cup ice cubes

Instructions:

1. Peel and slice the ripe bananas.
2. Place the sliced bananas, peanut butter, unsweetened almond milk, honey (optional), and vanilla extract, in a blender.
3. Add the ice cubes to the blender.
4. Blend everything until you get a smooth and creamy mixture.
5. Pour the smoothie into two glasses.
6. Serve and enjoy!

Nutritional Values per Person: Calories: 225 Protein: 6g Carbohydrates: 27g Fat: 11g Fiber: 4g

20. Greek Yogurt Parfait

Difficulty: Easy   Preparation Time: 10 minutes

Cooking Time: 0 minutes   Serving: 2

Ingredients:

- 1 cup non-fat Greek yogurt
- 1 tbsp. honey
- 1/2 tsp vanilla extract
- 1/2 cup fresh berries (such as strawberries, blueberries, raspberries)
- 1/4 cup granola
- 2 tbsp. chopped nuts (such as almonds, walnuts)

Instructions:

1. Combine the Greek yogurt, honey and vanilla extract in a mixing bowl.
2. Stir until the ingredients are well blended.
3. Wash and slice the fresh berries.
4. To assemble the parfaits, take two small cups or bowls and spoon a layer of the yogurt mixture onto the bottom of each.
5. Add a layer of sliced berries onto the yogurt in each cup.
6. Sprinkle a layer of granola on top of the berries in each cup.
7. Add another layer of the yogurt mixture on top of the granola in each cup.
8. Sprinkle a layer of chopped nuts on top of the yogurt in each cup.
9. Add a final layer of sliced berries on top of the nuts in each cup.
10. Serve and enjoy!

Nutritional Values per Person: Calories: 215 Protein: 16g Carbohydrates: 31g Fat: 5g Fiber: 4g

21. Quinoa Porridge with Dried Fruit

Difficulty: Easy   Preparation Time: 6 minutes

Cooking Time: 15 minutes Serving: 2

Ingredients:

- 1 cup uncooked quinoa
- 1 cup water
- 2 cups unsweetened almond milk x
- 1 tbsp. honey
- 1/4 tsp cinnamon
- 1/4 tsp salt
- 1/4 cup dried fruit (such as apricots, raisins or cranberries)
- 2 tbsp. chopped walnuts

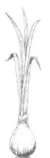

Instructions:

1. Rinse the quinoa with cold water and let it drain.
2. Turn the heat on to medium flame and bring the almond milk, quinoa and water to the boil in a saucepan. Cover the saucepan with a lid, lower the heat and cook for 15 minutes or until the liquid is absorbed and the quinoa is tender.
3. Stir in honey, cinnamon, and salt.
4. Add the dried fruit and stir for a minute until the fruit is plump and tender.
5. Divide the porridge into two bowls and sprinkle with chopped walnuts.
6. Serve warm.

Nutritional Values per Person: Calories: 383 Protein: 9.5 g Carbohydrates: 64.9 g Fat: 10.7 g Fiber: 7.3 g

22. Scrambled Eggs with Tomatoes and Spinach

Difficulty: Easy   Preparation Time: 6 minutes

Cooking Time: 12 minutes Serving: 2

Ingredients:

- 4 large eggs
- 1 medium tomato, diced
- 2 cups fresh spinach leaves
- 1 tbsp. olive oil
- Salt and pepper to taste

Instructions:

1. In a mixing bowl, beat the eggs until they are well mixed.
2. Turn the heat on to medium flame and heat a pan with the oil.
3. When the oil is hot, add the diced tomato and sauté for 3-4 minutes until it begins to soften.
4. Add the spinach leaves to the skillet and sauté for an additional 1-2 minutes until the spinach is wilted.
5. Pour the beaten eggs into the skillet and stir gently with a spatula.
6. Continue to stir the eggs until they are fully cooked, but still moist.
7. Season with salt and pepper.
8. Serve immediately.

Nutritional Values per Person: Calories: 223 Protein: 17g Carbohydrates: 6g Fat: 15g Fiber: 2g

23. Veggie and Cheese Omelet

Difficulty: Easy   Preparation Time: 10 minutes
Cooking Time: 10 minutes   Serving: 2
Ingredients:

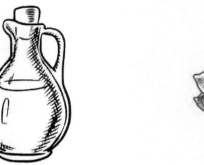
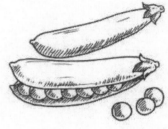

- 4 large eggs
- 1/4 cup chopped red bell pepper
- 1/4 cup chopped onion
- 1/4 cup sliced mushrooms
- 1/4 cup shredded cheddar cheese
- 1 tbsp. olive oil
- Salt and pepper to taste

Instructions:

1. In a mixing bowl, beat the eggs until they are well mixed.
2. Turn the heat to medium and add the oil to a pan.
3. Once the oil is hot, add the chopped bell pepper, onion, and sliced mushrooms to the skillet.
4. Sauté the vegetables for 3-4 minutes until they are tender.
5. Pour the beaten eggs into the skillet, tilting the pan to ensure that the eggs cover the entire surface of the skillet.
6. Allow the eggs to cook for 2-3 minutes until they are set on the bottom.
7. Sprinkle the cheddar cheese on one side of the omelette.
8. Gently fold in one side of the frit, with a spatula, forming a half moon.
9. Allow the cheese to melt for 1-2 minutes.
10. Slide the omelet onto a plate and season with salt and pepper.
11. Serve immediately.

Nutritional Values per Person: Calories: 296 Protein: 20g Carbohydrates: 5g Fat: 23g Fiber: 1g

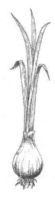

24. Low-Carb Blueberry Muffins

Difficulty: Easy   Preparation Time: 12 minutes
Cooking Time: 23 minutes   Serving: 12 muffins
Ingredients:

- 2 cups almond flour
- 1/2 cup granulated sweetener of choice
- 2 tsp baking powder
- 1/4 tsp salt
- 3 eggs
- 1/2 cup unsweetened almond milk
- 1/4 cup melted coconut oil
- 1 tsp vanilla extract
- 1 cup fresh blueberries

Instructions:

1. Heat the oven to 350°F and prepare a muffin pan with paper liners.
2. Combine almond flour, natural sweetener, baking powder, and salt in a mixing bowl.
3. In another bowl, mix eggs, almond milk, melted coconut oil, and vanilla extract.
4. Add the dry ingredients with the wet ingredients and mix until well blended.
5. Carefully add blueberries to the mixture and stir gently.
6. Pour the batter into the muffin liners, filling them to about 3/4 full.
7. Bake for nearly 25 minutes until the muffins are lightly browned and a thin wooden stick inserted in the center comes out clean.
8. Let the muffins cool in the pan for 12 minutes before transferring them to a cooling rack to cool completely.

Nutritional Values per Person: Calories: 139 Protein: 5g Carbohydrates: 5g Fat: 12g Fiber: 2g

25. Avocado Toast with Poached Egg

Difficulty: Easy   **Preparation Time:** 12 minutes

Cooking Time: 12 minutes   **Serving:** 2 servings

Ingredients:

- 2 slices of whole grain bread
- 1 ripe avocado
- 1 small garlic clove, minced
- 1/2 tsp lemon juice
- Salt and pepper
- 2 large eggs
- 1 tsp white vinegar

Instructions:

1. Toast the bread slices until crispy and golden brown.
2. While the bread is toasting, cut the avocado and remove the pit.
3. Scoop out the avocado flesh into a small mixing bowl.
4. Add the minced garlic, pepper, salt and lemon juice to the avocado.
5. Using a fork, mash the avocado until it's smooth and well combined with the other ingredients.
6. In a small saucepan, bring water to a simmer and add the vinegar.
7. Crack one egg into a small bowl.
8. Once the water is simmering, use a spoon to swirl the water in a circular motion.
9. Carefully pour the egg into the swirling water and let it cook for about 3-4 minutes.
10. Use a slotted spoon to remove the egg from the water and place it on a paper towel to remove any excess water.
11. Repeat with the second egg.
12. Spread the avocado mixture evenly onto the toasted bread slices.
13. Place one poached egg on each toast.
14. Sprinkle salt and pepper on top of the eggs as desired.

Nutritional Values per Person: Calories: 280 Protein: 13g Carbohydrates: 22g Fat: 18g Fiber: 10g

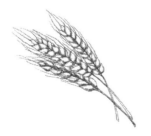

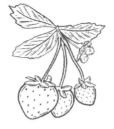

26. Spinach and Bacon Frittata

Difficulty: Easy   **Preparation Time:** 12 minutes

Cooking Time: 22 minutes   **Serving:** 4 servings

Ingredients:

- 6 large eggs
- 2 cups fresh spinach
- 3 slices of bacon
- 1/2 small onion, diced
- 1/2 tsp garlic powder
- Salt and pepper
- 1 tbsp. olive oil

Instructions:

1. Turn the oven on and bring it to 350°F (175°C).
2. In a mixing bowl, whisk together the eggs, garlic powder, pepper and salt.
3. Add the fresh spinach to the mixing bowl and gently stir to combine.
4. In a 10-inch oven-safe skillet, cook the bacon over medium-high heat until crispy.
5. Remove the cooked bacon from the pan and place it on a paper towel to remove any fat.
6. In the pan, add the diced onion and the olive oil.
7. Sauté the onion for about 3-4 minutes or until translucent.
8. Crumble the cooked bacon and add it to the skillet, along with the egg and spinach mixture.
9. Gently stir the mixture and cook on medium heat for about 5-7 minutes or until the edges start to set.
10. Place the skillet in the preheated oven and bake for about 8-10 minutes or until the frittata is fully cooked and golden brown on top.
11. Use a spatula to remove the frittata from the skillet and slice it into wedges.
12. Serve hot or at room temperature.

Nutritional Values per Person: Calories: 160 Protein: 10g Carbohydrates: 2g Fat: 12g Fiber: 1g

27. Breakfast Burrito

Difficulty: Easy   Preparation Time: 15 minutes
Cooking Time: 10 minutes Serving: 4 servings
Ingredients:

- 4 large flour tortillas
- 1/2 lb. ground turkey sausage
- 3 large eggs
- 1/2 small onion, diced
- 1 small bell pepper, diced Salt and pepper
- 1 tbsp. olive oil
- 1/2 cup shredded cheddar cheese
- 1 avocado, sliced
- 1/4 cup salsa

Instructions:

1. In a skillet, cook the turkey sausage over medium heat until browned and cooked through.
2. Remove the sausage from the pan and place it on a paper towel to remove any fat.
3. In the same pan, add the olive oil, bell pepper and diced onion.
4. Sauté the vegetables for about 3-4 minutes or until they are tender.
5. In a small mixing bowl, beat the eggs with salt and pepper.
6. Add the beaten eggs to the pan, stirring occasionally, until cooked through and scrambled.
7. Warm the flour tortillas in the oven or microwave.
8. Assemble the burritos by placing a scoop of the scrambled eggs, turkey sausage, shredded cheddar cheese, sliced avocado, and salsa.
9. Fold the sides of the tortilla inwards and then roll the burrito up tightly.
10. Serve the breakfast burritos hot.

Nutritional Values per Person: Calories: 420 Protein: 20g Carbohydrates: 25g Fat: 27g Fiber: 5g

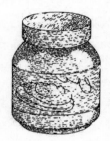

28. Coconut Quinoa Porridge with Fruit and Nuts

Difficulty: Easy   Preparation Time: 5 minutes
Cooking Time: 20 minutes Serving: 4 servings
Ingredients:

- 1 cup quinoa
- 1 can (13.5 oz.) coconut milk
- 1/2 cup water
- 2 tbsp. honey
- 1 tsp vanilla extract
- 1/2 tsp ground cinnamon
- 1/4 tsp salt
- 1/2 cup sliced fruit (banana, berries, or mango)
- 1/4 cup chopped nuts (almonds, walnuts, or pecans)

Instructions:

1. Rinse the quinoa in cold water and drain well.
2. In a saucepan, add the quinoa, water, coconut milk, honey, vanilla extract, ground cinnamon, and salt.
3. Bring a mixture to a boil over medium-high heat, stirring occasionally.
4. Reduce the heat to low and cover the pan with a lid.
5. Simmer the quinoa for 17 - 22 minutes until the quinoa is tender and the liquid is absorbed.
6. Turn off the heat and let the quinoa rest for 5 minutes.
7. Divide the quinoa porridge among 4 serving bowls.
8. Top each bowl with sliced fruit and chopped nuts.
9. Serve the coconut quinoa porridge warm.

Nutritional Values per Person: Calories: 360 Protein: 8g Carbohydrates: 38g Fat: 22g Fiber: 4g

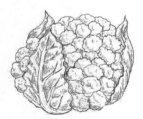

29. Sugar-free Oat and Banana Bars

Difficulty: Easy   Preparation Time: 10 minutes

Cooking Time: 30 minutes   Serving: 8 bars

Ingredients:

- 2 cups rolled oats
- 2 ripe bananas, mashed
- 1/4 cup unsweetened applesauce
- 1/4 cup almond butter
- 1 tsp vanilla extract
- 1 tsp ground cinnamon
- 1/4 tsp salt

- Optional add-ins: chopped nuts, raisins, chocolate chips (make sure they are no sugar added)

Instructions:

1. Turn the oven on and bring it to 350°F (180°C).
2. Line an 8x8 inch baking dish with parchment paper.
3. In a large bowl, mix together the oats, mashed bananas, unsweetened applesauce, almond butter, vanilla extract, ground cinnamon, and salt.
4. Add any optional add-ins of your choice.
5. Use a spoon to compact the mixture.
6. Bake the bars for 25-30 minutes or until they are lightly browned and firm to the touch.
7. Remove the pan from the oven and let the bars cool completely.
8. Use a sharp knife to cut the oat and banana bars into 8 evenly sized pieces.
9. Store the bars in a container in the refrigerator for up to 4 days.

Nutritional Values per Person: Calories: 180 Protein: 5g Carbohydrates: 25g Fat: 7g Fiber: 4g

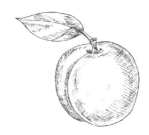

30. Healthy Pesto Pork Tenderloin Breakfast Bowl

Difficulty: Easy   Preparation Time: 12 minutes

Cooking Time: 20 minutes   Serving: 2 persons

Ingredients:

- 1/2 lb. pork tenderloin
- 1 tbsp. olive oil
- Salt and pepper to taste
- 1/4 cup prepared pesto
- 2 cups cooked brown rice
- 2 cups fresh spinach
- 1/2 avocado, sliced
- 1/4 cup cherry tomatoes, halved
- 2 tbsp. balsamic vinegar

Instructions:

1. Turn on the oven and bring it to 200°C and prepare a baking sheet with non-stick cooking spray.
2. Season the pork tenderloin with pepper and salt and place it in the baking dish.
3. Brush the pesto over the pork tenderloin, making sure to cover it completely.
4. Bake the pork for 19- 21 minutes or until it is cooked through.
5. While the pork is cooking, prepare the other ingredients. Cook the brown rice according to package instructions and wash the spinach leaves.
6. Once the pork is cooked, remove it from the oven and let it rest for 6-7 minutes, then cut it into thin pieces.
7. Divide the cooked brown rice into two bowls and top with fresh spinach leaves, sliced avocado, halved cherry tomatoes, and the sliced pesto pork tenderloin.
8. Drizzle each bowl with balsamic vinegar and serve hot.

Nutritional Values Per Person: Calories 438 Fat 21.2g Carbohydrates 37.4g Fiber 4.4g Protein 28.3g

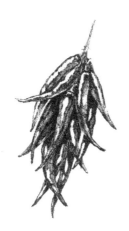

31. Sweet Potato Pancakes

Difficulty: Intermediate **Preparation Time:** 20 minutes
Cooking Time: 14 minutes **Serving:** 4
Ingredients:

- 1 medium sweet potato, peeled and grated
- 2 eggs
- 1/2 cup whole wheat flour
- 1/2 tsp baking powder
- 1/2 tsp cinnamon
- 1/4 tsp salt
- 2 tbsp. honey
- 1 tbsp. coconut oil
- Optional toppings: Greek yogurt, sliced bananas, chopped nuts

Instructions:

1. In a bowl, mix together the grated sweet potato and eggs.
2. In a separate bowl, combine the whole wheat flour, cinnamon, baking powder, and salt.
3. Gradually add the dry ingredients to the sweet potato mixture, stirring until well combined.
4. Add the honey and mix until evenly distributed.
5. Melt the coconut oil in a large skillet over medium heat.
6. Spoon about 2 tbsp. of batter onto the skillet for each pancake.
7. Cook for 2-3 minutes on each side, or until golden brown.
8. Repeat until all of the batter has been used.
9. Top the pancakes with Greek yogurt, sliced bananas, and chopped nuts, if desired.

Nutritional Values per Person: Calories: 230 Protein: 8g Carbohydrates: 36g Fat: 7g Fiber: 5g

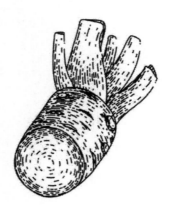

32. Matcha Tea Smoothie Bowl

Difficulty: Easy **Preparation Time:** 10 minutes
Cooking Time: 0 minutes **Serving:** 2
Ingredients:

- 2 bananas, sliced and frozen
- 1 tsp matcha tea powder
- 1/2 cup almond milk
- 1/2 cup Greek yogurt
- 1 tbsp. honey
- 1/4 cup granola
- 1/4 cup sliced strawberries
- 1 tbsp. chia seeds

Instructions:

1. In a blender, combine the frozen bananas, matcha tea powder, almond milk, Greek yogurt, and honey.
2. Blend until smooth and creamy.
3. Pour the mixture into two bowls.
4. Add the granola, sliced strawberries, and chia seeds on top of the smoothie mixture.
5. Serve immediately and enjoy!

Nutritional Values per Person: Calories: 285 Protein: 12g Carbohydrates: 50g Fat: 6g Fiber: 8g

Snacks

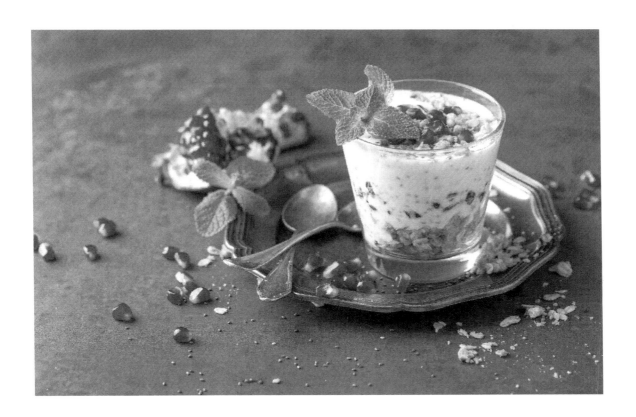

33. Avocado and Cottage Cheese Toast

Difficulty: Easy **Preparation Time:** 10 minutes

Cooking Time: 5 minutes **Serving:** 2

Ingredients:

- 2 slices of whole grain bread, toasted
- 1 ripe avocado, sliced
- 1/2 cup low-fat cottage cheese
- 1/2 tsp garlic powder
- Salt and black pepper
- 1 small tomato, sliced
- 2 tbsp. chopped fresh parsley

Instructions:

1. In a small bowl, mix the cottage cheese, garlic powder, black pepper and salt.
2. Spread the cottage cheese mixture evenly on the toasted bread slices.
3. Layer the sliced avocado and tomato on top of the cottage cheese mixture.
4. Sprinkle freshly chopped parsley on top of each slice.
5. Serve immediately and enjoy!

Nutritional Values per Person: Calories: 250 Protein: 15g Carbohydrates: 25g Fat: 10g Fiber: 8g

34. Baked Sweet Potato Chips

Difficulty: Easy **Preparation Time:** 10 minutes

Cooking Time: 15-20 minutes **Serving:** 2-3

Ingredients:

- 2 medium-sized sweet potatoes, peeled and sliced into thin rounds
- 1 tbsp. olive oil
- 1/2 tsp sea salt
- 1/2 tsp smoked paprika
- Optional: additional spices such as garlic powder, onion powder, or chili powder

Instructions:

1. Turn the oven on and bring it to 375°F (190°C).
2. In a bowl, toss the sweet potato wedges with the olive oil and spices until well coated.
3. Arrange the sweet potato wedges in one layer on a parchment-lined baking sheet.
4. Bake for 15-20 minutes, flipping the chips halfway through, until the edges are crispy and slightly browned.
5. Remove from the oven and let cool before serving.

Nutritional Values per Person: Calories: 150 Protein: 2g Carbohydrates: 23g Fat: 6g Fiber: 4g

35. Greek Yogurt and Berries

Difficulty: Easy **Preparation Time:** 6 minutes

Cooking Time: 0 minutes **Serving:** 1

Ingredients:

- 1 cup plain Greek yogurt
- 1/2 cup mixed berries (such as blueberries, raspberries, and strawberries)
- 1 tbsp. honey
- Optional toppings: sliced almonds, chia seeds, or granola

Instructions:

1. In a small bowl, mix together the Greek yogurt and honey until well combined.
2. Wash the mixed berries and chop them if necessary.
3. Spoon the yogurt mixture into a serving bowl or glass.
4. Top the yogurt with the mixed berries and any additional toppings of your choice.
5. Serve immediately or store in the refrigerator for later.

Nutritional Values per Person: Calories: 250 Protein: 21g Carbohydrates: 37g Fat: 3g Fiber: 5g

36. Tuna Salad and Cucumber Slices

Difficulty: Easy **Preparation Time:** 10 minutes

Cooking Time: 0 minutes **Serving:** 2

Ingredients:

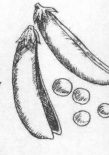

- 1 can of tuna, drained
- 1/4 cup diced red onion
- 1/4 cup diced celery
- 1 tbsp. finely chopped fresh parsley
- 1 tbsp. lemon juice
- 2 tbsp. olive oil
- Salt and pepper, to taste
- 1 large cucumber, washed and sliced into rounds

Instructions:

1. In a small bowl, combine the drained tuna, diced red onion, diced celery, chopped fresh parsley, olive oil, and lemon juice. Mix well.
2. Season the tuna salad with salt and pepper to taste.
3. Wash and slice the cucumber into rounds.
4. Serve the tuna salad on top of the cucumber slices.

Nutritional Values per Person: Calories: 240 Protein: 22g Carbohydrates: 6g Fat: 15g Fiber: 1.5g

37. Roasted Chickpeas

Difficulty: Easy   **Preparation Time:** 11 minutes

Cooking Time: 40 minutes   **Serving:** 4

Ingredients:

- 2 cans of chickpeas, drained and rinsed
- 2 tbsp. olive oil
- 1/2 tsp garlic powder
- 1/2 tsp cumin
- 1/2 tsp paprika
- 1/2 tsp salt

Instructions:

1. Turn the oven on and bring it to 375°F (190°C).
2. Drain and rinse the chickpeas.
3. Spread the chickpeas onto a paper towel and pat dry to remove excess water.
4. Transfer the chickpeas to a mixing bowl.
5. Add the olive oil, garlic powder, cumin, salt and paprika to the mixing bowl. Toss until the chickpeas are evenly coated.
6. In a pan with baking paper and arrange the chickpeas in one layer.
7. Roast the chickpeas in the oven for 30-40 minutes or until golden brown and crispy.
8. Remove the baking sheet from the oven and let the chickpeas cool for 6 minutes before serving.

Nutritional Values per Person: Calories: 175 Protein: 6g Carbohydrates: 19g Fat: 8g Fiber: 6g

38. Mediterranean Hummus Dip with Veggies

Difficulty: Easy   **Preparation Time:** 12 minutes

Cooking Time: None   **Serving:** 4

Ingredients:

- 1 can of chickpeas, drained and rinsed1/4 cup tahini
- 1/4 cup lemon juice
- 2 cloves of garlic, minced
- 1/2 tsp ground cumin
- 1/2 tsp paprika
- 1/4 tsp salt
- Assorted vegetables (carrots, cucumber, bell peppers, etc.) for dipping

Instructions:

1. Drain and rinse the chickpeas.
2. In a food processor, combine the chickpeas, lemon juice, tahini, garlic, cumin, paprika, and salt.
3. Process the mixture until it becomes a smooth texture.

4. Taste the hummus and adjust the seasoning as needed.
5. Transfer the hummus to a serving bowl.
6. Wash and chop the assorted vegetables into bite-sized pieces.
7. Arrange the vegetables around the hummus dip in a platter or tray.
8. Serve and enjoy!

Nutritional Values per Person: Calories: 160 Protein: 8g Carbohydrates: 16g Fat: 8g Fiber: 6g

39. Spinach Stuffed Mushrooms

Difficulty: Intermediate   **Preparation Time:** 25 minutes

Cooking Time: 22 minutes   **Serving:** 4

Ingredients:

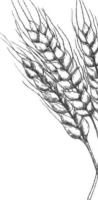

- 24 large mushrooms, stemmed
- 3 tbsp. olive oil
- 1 onion, chopped
- 2 cloves garlic, minced
- 8 ounces fresh spinach, chopped
- 1/4 cup breadcrumbs
- 1/4 cup grated Parmesan cheese
- 1/2 tsp salt
- 1/4 tsp black pepper

Instructions:

1. Turn the oven on and turn it to 375°F.
2. Remove the mushroom stems and rinse them.
3. Heat 2 tablespoons of oil in a large skillet.
4. Add the garlic and onion and cook them for about 5 minutes until soft.
5. Add the chopped spinach and cook until wilted, about 3-4 minutes.
6. Remove from heat and add the breadcrumbs, Parmesan cheese, pepper and salt. Stir well.
7. Using a small spoon, fill each mushroom cap with the spinach mixture and place them on a greased baking sheet.
8. Drizzle each mushroom with the remaining olive oil.
9. Cook until the mushrooms are tender, about 20 minutes.
10. Serve hot and enjoy!

Nutritional Values per Person: Calories: 130 Protein: 6g Carbohydrates: 8g Fat: 9g Fiber: 2g

40. Healthy Omega-3 Bagel

Difficulty: Easy   **Preparation Time:** 12 minutes
Cooking Time: 3-5 minutes (toasting the bagel) **Serving:** 1
Ingredients:

- 1 whole grain bagel
- 2 oz. smoked salmon
- 1 tbsp. low-fat cream cheese
- 1 tsp fresh squeezed lemon juice
- 1/2 small cucumber, sliced
- 1/4 small red onion, sliced
- 1/4 small avocado, sliced
- Salt and black pepper

Instructions:

1. Toast the whole grain bagel until it's slightly crispy.
2. In a small bowl, mix the low-fat cream cheese and lemon juice until smooth. Spread the cream cheese mixture on one half of the bagel.
3. Lay the smoked salmon on top of the cream cheese mixture.
4. Top the smoked salmon with sliced cucumber, red onion, and avocado. Add salt and black pepper.
5. Cover with the other half of the bagel and serve.

Nutritional Values per Person: Calories: 367 Protein: 23.2 g Carbohydrates: 38.6 g Fat: 15.8 g Fiber: 7.2 g

41. Crunchy Mozzarella Cauliflower

Difficulty: Easy   **Preparation Time:** 15 minutes
Cooking Time: 40 minutes   **Servings:** 12
Ingredients:

- 1 large cauliflower head, riced
- 1 cup low-fat mozzarella cheese, shredded
- ¼ cup all-purpose flour
- 2 eggs
- 1 tsp Italian seasoning
- 1/2 tsp garlic powder
- 1/2 tsp onion powder
- 1/2 tsp paprika
- Salt and black pepper to taste
- Cooking spray

Instructions:

1. Turn on the oven and bring it to 190°C (375°F). Line a baking sheet with parchment paper and spray with cooking spray.
2. Spread the cauliflower rice on the lined baking sheet, and bake for 20 minutes.

3. Transfer the cauliflower rice to a bowl and set aside to cool for a few minutes.
4. Add the mozzarella cheese, flour, eggs, Italian seasoning, garlic powder, onion powder, paprika, black pepper and salt to the cauliflower rice, and mix well.
5. Spread the mixture into a rectangular pan and press down to create an even surface.
6. Bake the cauliflower bites in the oven for 20 minutes, or until golden brown.
7. Remove the tray from the oven and leave to cool. Cut into 12 equal bars.
8. Serve these Crunchy Mozzarella Cauliflower Bites hot as a snack, or with your favorite dip.

Nutritional Values per Person: Calories 100 Kcal Fat: 4g Carbohydrates: 7g Protein: 7g.

42. Hummus with Carrots and Cucumber

Difficulty: Easy   **Preparation Time:** 12 minutes
Cooking Time: 0 minutes   **Serving:** 4
Ingredients:

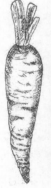

- 1 can (15 oz.) chickpeas, drained and rinsed
- 3 tbsp. tahini
- 3 tbsp. extra-virgin olive oil
- 3 tbsp. lemon juice
- 1 garlic clove, minced
- 1/2 tsp ground cumin
- Salt and pepper
- 2 medium carrots, peeled and chopped
- 1 medium cucumber, chopped

Instructions:

1. In a blender or food processor, combine the chickpeas, tahini, lemon juice, olive oil, garlic, cumin, salt, and pepper. Process until smooth, gradually adding a little water as needed to achieve desired consistency.
2. Transfer the hummus to a serving bowl and top with chopped carrots and cucumber.
3. Serve immediately with pita chips or other dipping veggies.

Nutritional Values per Person: Calories: 210 Protein: 8g Carbohydrates: 19g Fat: 12g Fiber: 6g

43. Broccoli Bites

Difficulty: Easy   **Preparation Time:** 10 minutes

Cooking Time: 22 minutes   **Serving:** 4

Ingredients:

- 1 head of broccoli, cut into small florets
- 2 tbsp. olive oil
- 1/4 cup whole wheat flour
- 1/4 cup grated Parmesan cheese
- 1/4 tsp garlic powder
- Salt and pepper
- 1 egg, lightly beaten
- Cooking spray

Instructions:

1. Turn on the oven and bring it to 375°F (190°C).
2. In a mixing bowl, combine the flour, Parmesan cheese, salt, garlic powder and pepper.
3. Add the broccoli florets to the bowl and mix until the florets are coated in the flour mixture.
4. Dip each broccoli floret into the beaten egg mixture, shaking off any excess.
5. Arrange the coated broccoli florets on a baking sheet with parchment paper.
6. Lightly spray the broccoli florets with cooking spray.
7. Bake the broccoli poppers in the oven for 22-27 minutes until they turn crispy and golden brown.
8. Once done, remove the baking sheet from the oven and let cool for 5 minutes.
9. Transfer the roasted broccoli poppers to a serving bowl and serve as a healthy snack.

Nutritional Values per Serving: **Calories:** 130 **Fat:** 8g **Carbohydrates:** 11g **Fiber:** 4g **Protein:** 6g

44. Mexican Stuffed Bell Peppers

Difficulty: Medium   **Preparation Time:** 20 minutes

Cooking Time: 45 minutes   **Serving:** 4

Ingredients:

- 4 bell peppers, tops removed and seeds removed
- 1 lb. lean ground beef
- 1 small onion, diced
- 2 cloves garlic, minced
- 1 cup cooked brown rice
- 1/2 cup tomato sauce
- 1 tsp Italian seasoning
- Salt and pepper
- Optional toppings: shredded cheese, chopped parsley

Instructions:

1. Turn the oven on and turn it up to 350°F.
2. Brown the ground beef with the diced onion and minced garlic in a pan over medium heat.
3. Stir in the cooked brown rice, tomato sauce, Italian seasoning, and some salt and pepper.
4. Stuff each of the bell peppers with the meat and rice mixture.
5. Place the stuffed peppers in a baking dish, and cover with foil.
6. After baking 40 minutes, remove the foil and sprinkle with grated cheese if desired.
7. Bake for an additional 5-10 minutes, until the cheese is melted and bubbly.
8. Serve the stuffed peppers hot, and enjoy!

Nutritional Values per Person: Calories: 346 **Protein:** 26g **Carbohydrates:** 23g **Fat:** 16g **Fiber:** 5g

45. Roasted Beet and Goat Cheese Salad

Difficulty: Easy   **Preparation Time:** 10 minutes

Cooking Time: 45 minutes   **Serving:** 4

Ingredients:

- 4 medium-sized beets, washed, peeled, and cut into wedges
- 2 tbsp. extra-virgin olive oilSalt and pepper
- 4 cups mixed greens
- 4 oz. crumbled goat cheese
- 1/4 cup chopped toasted walnuts
- 2 tbsp. balsamic vinegar
- 2 tbsp. honey

Instructions:

1. Turn the oven on and turn it to 375°F.
2. Season the beetroot slices with pepper, olive oil and salt.
3. Arrange the beets on a baking sheet and roast them for 40 minutes, stirring halfway through cooking.
4. Whisk together the honey and balsamic vinegar in a bowl to make the dressing.
5. Divide the mixed greens among 4 plates.
6. Top the greens with the roasted beets, crumbled goat cheese, and chopped walnuts.
7. Drizzle the balsamic dressing over the salad.
8. Serve the roasted beet and goat cheese salad immediately, and enjoy!

Nutritional Values per Person: Calories: 280 **Protein:** 9g **Carbohydrates:** 23g **Fat:** 19g **Fiber:** 5g

46. Broiled Grapefruit with Honey and Cinnamon

Difficulty: Easy   **Preparation Time:** 6 minutes
Cooking Time: 5 minutes   **Serving:** 2

Ingredients:

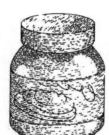

- 1 large grapefruit
- 2 tbsp. honey
- 1 tsp ground cinnamon

Instructions:

1. Preheat the broiler.
2. Cut the grapefruit in half crosswise and use a small knife to loosen the segments from the membrane.
3. Place the grapefruit halves on a baking sheet.
4. Drizzle the honey over each half and sprinkle the cinnamon on top.
5. Broil the grapefruit for 5 minutes, or until the topping is bubbly and lightly browned.
6. Remove the grapefruit from the oven and let it cool.
7. Serve the broiled grapefruit halves immediately and enjoy!

Nutritional Values per Person: Calories: 90 Protein: 1g Carbohydrates: 24g Fat: 0g Fiber: 2g

47. Oatmeal Raisin Cookies

Difficulty: Easy   **Preparation Time:** 17 minutes
Cooking Time: 13-16 minutes   **Serving:** 12-15 cookies

Ingredients:

- 1/2 cup unsalted butter, softened
- 1/2 cup brown sugar
- 1/4 cup granulated sugar
- 1 egg
- 1 tsp vanilla extract
- 1 cup all-purpose flour
- 1/2 tsp baking soda
- 1/2 tsp salt
- 1 1/2 cups old-fashioned oats
- 3/4 cups raisins

Instructions:

1. Bring the oven to 180°C and line a baking tray with baking paper.
2. In a large mixing bowl, cream the softened butter with the brown sugar and granulated sugar.
3. Blend the mixture by adding the vanilla extract and the egg.
4. Add and mix well in another bowl the baking soda, flour and salt, and gradually fold the flour mixture into the wet mixture mixing well.
5. Add the old-fashioned oats and raisins into the bowl and stir to combine.

6. Take small portions of the dough and roll them into balls. Place them about two inches apart on the prepared baking sheet.
7. Flatten each ball slightly with your hand or the back of a spoon.
8. Bake for 12-15 minutes, or until lightly browned.
9. Allow to cool before removing from the baking sheet.

Nutritional Values per Person:

- Calories: 170
- Protein: 2g
- Carbohydrates: 24g
- Fat: 7g
- Fiber: 1g

48. Lemon and Ginger Cookies

Difficulty: Easy   **Preparation Time:** 16 minutes
Cooking Time: 12-15 minutes   **Serving:** 13-16 cookies

Ingredients:

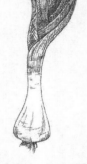

- -1/2 cup unsalted butter, softened
- -1/2 cup granulated sugar
- -1 egg
- -1 tbsp. grated fresh ginger
- -1 tbsp. lemon zest
- -1 1/2 cup all-purpose flour
- -1/2 tsp baking powder
- -1/4 tsp salt

Instructions:

1. Bring the oven to 180°C and line a baking tray with baking paper.
2. In a large mixing bowl, cream the softened butter and granulated sugar together until light and fluffy.
3. beat in the egg, grated ginger, and lemon zest.
4. In a separate bowl, whisk together the flour, salt, and baking powder.
5. Gradually stir the flour mixture into the butter mixture and blend well.
6. Roll the dough into a log shape, wrap it in plastic wrap, and refrigerate for 30 minutes.
7. Remove the dough from the refrigerator and slice into 1/4 inch rounds.
8. Place the rounds on the prepared baking sheet and bake for 12-15 minutes or until lightly golden.
9. Remove from the oven and cool on a wire rack.

Nutritional Values per Person: Calories: 140 Protein: 2g Carbohydrates: 16g Fat: 8g Fiber: 0.5g

49. Peanut Butter and Banana Cookies

Difficulty: Easy   **Preparation Time:** 20 minutes

Cooking Time: 10-12 minutes   **Serving:** 12-15 cookies

Ingredients:

- 1/2 cup unsalted butter, melted
- 1/2 cup brown sugar
- 1/4 cup granulated sugar
- 1 egg
- 1 ripe banana, mashed
- 1 cup creamy peanut butter
- 1/2 tsp vanilla extract
- 1 1/2 cups all-purpose flour
- 1/2 tsp baking powder
- 1/2 tsp baking soda
- 1/2 tsp salt

Instructions:

1. Bring the oven to 180°C and line a baking tray with parchment paper.

2. In a mixing bowl, combine the melted butter with the brown sugar and granulated sugar until smooth.

3. Add the egg, mashed banana, creamy peanut butter and vanilla extract to the mixture and whisk well.

4. Add and mix well in another bowl the baking soda, flour and salt, and gradually fold the flour mixture into the wet mixture mixing well.

5. Using a cookie scoop or your hands, form small balls of dough and place them roughly two inches apart on the baking sheet. Flatten them gently with a fork, creating a crisscross pattern.

6. Bake for 10-12 minutes or until the edges begin to turn golden. Allow to cool before removing from the baking sheet.

Nutritional Values per Person: Calories: 220 Protein: 6g Carbohydrates: 21gFat: 14g Fiber: 2g

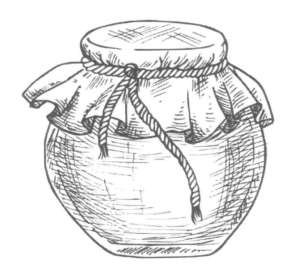

Beans, Cereals, Pasta, Rice

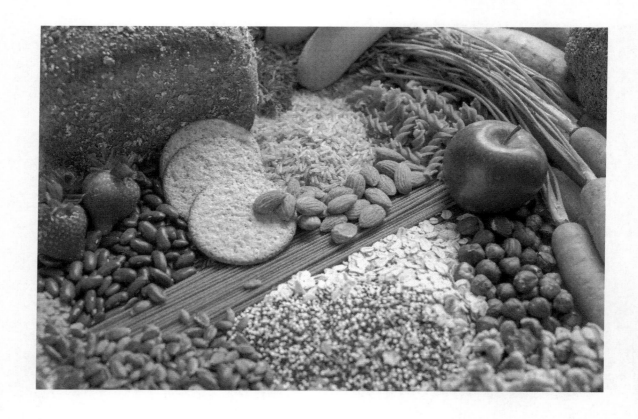

50. Mixed Vegetable Lentil Soup

Difficulty: Easy **Preparation Time:** 12 minutes

Cooking Time: 45 minutes **Serving:** 4

Ingredients:

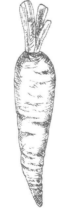

- 1 tbsp. olive oil
- 1 onion, chopped
- 2 garlic cloves, minced
- 2 carrots, peeled and chopped
- 2 celery stalks, chopped
- 1 zucchini, chopped
- 1 can (14 oz.) diced tomatoes
- 1 cup green or brown lentils
- 6 cups low-sodium vegetable broth
- 1 tsp ground cumin
- 1/2 tsp smoked paprika
- Salt and black pepper
- 2 tbsp. chopped fresh parsley

Instructions:

1. Heat the oil in a saucepan over medium heat. Add garlic and onion and sauté for about 6 minutes.
2. Add the courgettes, carrots and celery and continue to cook for another 6 minutes.
3. Add the diced tomatoes, lentils, cumin, salt, pepper, paprika and vegetable stock. Bring to the boil.
4. Put the lid on, reduce the heat and simmer, until the vegetables and lentils are tender, about 30-35 minutes.
5. Stir in the chopped parsley and serve.

Nutritional Values per Person: **Calories: 296 Fat: 4.7g Carbohydrates: 50.2g Fiber: 22.2g Protein: 17.3g**

51. Chickpea Salad with Radishes and Carrots

Difficulty: Easy **Preparation Time:** 12 minutes

Cooking Time: None **Serving:** 4

Ingredients:

- 2 cans (15 oz.) chickpeas, drained and rinsed
- 4 radishes, thinly sliced
- 2 carrots, peeled and grated
- 1/4 cup chopped fresh parsley
- 1/4 cup chopped fresh mint
- 2 tbsps. lemon juice
- 2 tbsps. extra-virgin olive oil
- Salt and black pepper

Instructions:

1. In a large bowl, combine the chickpeas, radishes, carrots, parsley, and mint.
2. In a bowl, whisk together the oil, salt, black pepper and the lemon juice.
3. Pour the dressing over the chickpea mixture and toss to coat.
4. Serve immediately or refrigerate until ready to serve.

Nutritional Values per Person: Calories: 255 Fat: 10.7g Carbohydrates: 29.1g Fiber: 10.4g Protein: 10.8g

52. Bean and Vegetable Curry

Difficulty: Easy **Preparation Time:** 15 minutes

Cooking Time: 30 minutes **Serving:** 4

Ingredients:

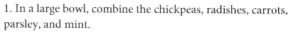

- 1 tbsp. olive oil
- 1 onion, diced
- 2 cloves garlic, minced
- 1 tbsp. grated ginger
- 1 tbsp. curry powder
- 1/2 tsp ground cumin
- 1/2 tsp ground coriander
- 1/4 tsp turmeric
- 1 can (14.5 oz.) diced tomatoes
- 1 can (15 oz.) kidney beans, drained and rinsed
- 2 cups mixed vegetables (such as zucchini, carrots, and green beans), chopped
- 1/2 cup water
- Salt and black pepper

Instructions:

1. In a Dutch oven or large pot, heat the olive oil over medium heat.
2. Add the garlic and onion and sauté for 3-4 minutes, until softened.
3. Add the ginger, curry powder, cumin, coriander, and turmeric and stir to combine.
4. Add the tomatoes and their juices, the kidney beans, mixed vegetables, and water. Stir to combine.
5. Bring to a boil and cook for 20-25 minutes, until vegetables are tender.
6. Season with salt and black pepper.
7. Serve immediately over steamed rice or with naan bread.

Nutritional Values per Person: Calories: 205 Fat: 4.8g Carbohydrates: 33.7g Fiber: 10.8g Protein: 9.1g

53. Mixed Bean and Vegetable Soup

Difficulty: Easy **Preparation Time:** 15 minutes

Cooking Time: 1 hour and 30 minutes **Serving:** 6

Ingredients:

- 1 tbsp. olive oil
- 1 onion, diced
- 2 cloves garlic, minced
- 2 carrots, diced
- 2 stalks celery, diced
- 1 can (14.5 oz.) diced tomatoes
- 1 can (15 oz.) mixed beans, drained and rinsed
- 6 cups vegetable broth
- 2 bay leaves
- 1/2 tsp dried thyme
- Salt and black pepper
- 2 cups mixed vegetables (such as potatoes, green beans, and squash), chopped
- 1/2 cup chopped fresh parsley

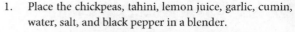

Instructions:

1. In a large saucepan, heat the olive oil over medium heat.
2. Add the garlic and onion and sauté for 4 minutes.
3. Add the celery and carrots and cook for about 6 minutes
4. Add the diced tomatoes, mixed beans, vegetable broth, bay leaves, thyme, black pepper and salt. Stir to combine.
5. Bring the soup to a boil, turn the heat down to low and cook for 30-45 minutes.
6. Add the mixed vegetables and continue to simmer for an additional 30 minutes, or until all the vegetables are tender.
7. Remove the bay leaves and season the soup with additional pepper and salt.
8. Stir in the chopped parsley and serve hot.

Nutritional Values per Person: Calories: 212 Fat: 3.6g Carbohydrates: 36.2g Fiber: 11.6g Protein: 11.1g

54. Chickpea Hummus

Difficulty: Easy **Preparation Time:** 12 minutes

Cooking Time: None **Serving:** 6

Ingredients:

- 2 cans (15 oz. each) chickpeas, drained and rinsed
- 1/4 cup tahini
- 1/4 cup freshly squeezed lemon juice
- 2 cloves garlic, minced
- 1/2 tsp ground cumin
- 1/4 cup water
- Salt and black pepper
- Paprika and olive oil for garnish

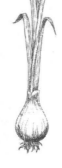

Instructions:

1. Place the chickpeas, tahini, lemon juice, garlic, cumin, water, salt, and black pepper in a blender.
2. Process the mixture on high speed for 1-2 minutes, or until smooth and creamy.
3. Taste the hummus and adjust the seasoning with additional salt and pepper if needed.
4. Serve the hummus in a bowl, sprinkled with paprika and drizzled with olive oil.

Nutritional Values per Person: Calories: 172 Fat: 9.9g Carbohydrates: 17.6g Fiber: 4.3g Protein: 6.1g

55. Brown Rice Pilaf with Spinach

Difficulty: Easy **Preparation Time:** 10 minutes

Cooking Time: 40 minutes **Serving:** 4

Ingredients:

- 1 cup brown rice
- 2 cups water
- 2 tbsps. olive oil
- 1 onion, chopped
- 2 cloves garlic, minced
- 1 tsp dried thyme
- 1/2 tsp salt
- 1/4 tsp black pepper
- 2 cups fresh spinach, chopped
- 1/4 cup toasted slivered almonds

Instructions:

1. Rinse the brown rice and drain well.
2. In a saucepan put the rice with the water and bring to a boil over high heat.
3. Reduce the heat to low and cover the pot, cooking the rice for 35-40 minutes, or until tender and the water has absorbed.
4. While the rice is cooking, heat the olive oil in a large skillet over medium heat.
5. Add the onion to the pan and cook for 5-6 minutes.
6. Add the garlic, thyme, salt, and black pepper to the skillet, and cook for an additional 1-2 minutes.
7. Aggiungere gli spinaci nella padella e cuocere per circa 2-3 minuti.
8. Once the rice has finished cooking, add it to the skillet with the spinach mixture and stir to combine.
9. Toast the slivered almonds in a dry skillet over low heat for 3-4 minutes, or until golden brown.
10. Sprinkle the toasted almonds over the rice pilaf just before serving.

Nutritional Values per Person: Calories: 272 Fat: 11g Carbohydrates: 38g Fiber: 4g Protein: 7g

56. Wild Rice Salad with Broccoli

Difficulty: Easy   **Preparation Time:** 15 minutes

Cooking Time: 45 minutes   **Serving:** 4

Ingredients:

- 1 cup wild rice
- 2 cups water
- 4 cups broccoli florets
- 1/2 cup dried cranberries
- 1/2 cup chopped pecans
- 1/4 cup chopped fresh parsley
- 1/4 cup olive oil
- 2 tbsps. apple cider vinegar
- 1 tbsp. honey
- 1 tsp Dijon mustard
- Salt and pepper to taste

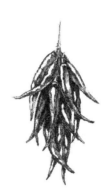

Instructions:

1. Rinse the wild rice and drain well.
2. In a pot, add the rice and water, and bring to a boil over high heat.
3. Reduce the heat to low and cover the pot, simmering the rice for 40-45 minutes, or until tender and most of the water has been absorbed.
4. While the rice is cooking, steam the broccoli florets over boiling water for 3-4 minutes, or until tender but still firm.
5. Once the rice has finished cooking, allow it to cool for 5-10 minutes.
6. In a large mixing bowl, combine the cooled rice, steamed broccoli, dried cranberries, chopped pecans, and fresh parsley.
7. In a small mixing bowl, whisk together the olive oil, apple cider vinegar, honey, Dijon mustard, salt, and pepper.
8. Pour the dressing over the rice and broccoli mixture, and toss gently to combine.
9. Cool the salad and serve.

Nutritional Values per Person: Calories: 355 **Fat:** 22g **Carbohydrates:** 38g **Fiber:** 6g **Protein:** 7g

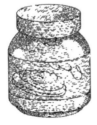

57. Brown Basmati Rice Salad with Peppers and Almonds

Difficulty: Easy   **Preparation Time:** 15 minutes

Cooking Time: 40 minutes   **Serving:** 4

Ingredients:

- 1 cup brown basmati rice
- 2 cups water
- 1 red bell pepper, diced
- 1 yellow bell pepper, diced
- 1/2 cup sliced almonds
- 2 green onions, thinly sliced
- 2 tbsps. olive oil
- 2 tbsps. lemon juice
- 1 tbsp. honey
- 1 tsp Dijon mustard
- Salt and pepper to taste

Instructions:

1. Rinse the brown basmati rice and drain well.
2. Place the rice and water in a pot and bring to a boil over high heat.
3. Reduce the heat to low and cover the pot, simmering the rice for 35-40 minutes, or until tender and most of the water has been absorbed.
4. While the rice is cooking, dice the red and yellow pepper, slice the almonds, and thinly slice the green onions.
5. Once the rice has finished cooking, allow it to cool for 5-10 minutes.
6. In a large mixing bowl, combine the cooled rice, diced peppers, sliced almonds, and green onions.
7. Whisk together the lemon juice, olive oil, honey, Dijon mustard, pepper and salt in a small saucepan.
8. Pour the dressing over the rice and pepper mixture, and toss gently to combine.
9. Let the salad cool and serve.

Nutritional Values per Person: Calories: 270 **Fat:** 12g **Carbohydrates:** 35g **Fiber:** 4g **Protein:** 6g

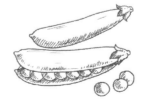

58. Brown Basmati Rice with Squash and Walnuts

Difficulty: Easy   **Preparation Time:** 20 minutes

Cooking Time: 50 minutes   **Serving:** 4

Ingredients:

- 1 cup brown basmati rice
- 2 cups water
- 1 small butternut squash, peeled and cut into small cubes
- 1/2 cup chopped walnuts
- 1/4 cup chopped parsley
- 2 tbsps. olive oil
- 1 tbsp. honey
- 1 tbsp. balsamic vinegar
- Salt and pepper

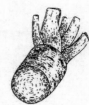

Instructions:

1. Rinse the brown basmati rice and drain well.
2. In a pot, add the rice and water and bring to a boil over high heat.
3. Reduce the heat to low and cover the pot, simmering the rice for 35-40 minutes, or until tender and most of the water has been absorbed.
4. Meanwhile, heat the olive oil in a saucepan over medium heat.
5. Add the cubed butternut squash and cook, stirring occasionally, until they start to caramelize, about 10-15 minutes.
6. Turn the oven on and bring it to 350°F.
7. Spread the chopped walnuts on a baking sheet and toast them in the oven for 5-7 minutes.
8. Once the rice has finished cooking, add the cooked squash, toasted walnuts, and chopped parsley to the pot.
9. In a small mixing bowl, whisk together the olive oil, honey, balsamic vinegar, pepper and salt.
10. Pour the dressing over the rice and vegetable mixture and toss gently to combine.
11. Serve immediately.

Nutritional Values per Person: Calories: 380 Fat: 19g Carbohydrates: 47g Fiber: 6g Protein: 8g

59. Wild Rice and Mushroom Pilaf

Difficulty: Medium   **Preparation Time:** 15 minutes

Cooking Time: 1 hour 15 minutes   **Serving:** 6

Ingredients:

- 1 cup wild rice
- 2 1/2 cups water or vegetable broth
- 1 tbsp. olive oil
- 1 onion, chopped
- 3 garlic cloves, minced
- 1 pound mushrooms, sliced
- 1/4 cup chopped fresh parsley
- 1/4 cup slivered almonds, toasted
- Salt and pepper to taste

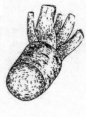

Instructions:

1. Turn the oven on and bring it to 350°F.
2. Rinse the wild rice in cold water and drain well.
3. In a pot, add the wild rice and water or vegetable broth and bring to a boil over high heat.
4. Reduce the heat to low and cover the pot, simmering the rice for 1 hour, or until tender and most of the water has been absorbed.
5. In the meantime, in a pan, heat olive oil over medium heat.
6. Add the chopped onion and garlic and cook until they start to soften, about 5 minutes.
7. Add the sliced mushrooms and cook until they start to release their liquid and become tender, about 10-15 minutes.
8. Once the wild rice has finished cooking, add the cooked mushroom mixture, chopped parsley, and slivered almonds to the pot.
9. Season with salt and pepper to taste and mix gently.
10. Transfer the mixture to an oven-safe dish and bake in the preheated oven for 15-20 minutes to let the flavors meld together.
11. Serve hot.

Nutritional Values per Person: Calories: 175 Fat: 5g Carbohydrates: 28g Fiber: 4g Protein: 7g

60. Brown Basmati Rice and Lentil Soup

Difficulty: Easy   **Preparation Time:** 15 minutes

Cooking Time: 45 minutes   **Serving:** 4

Ingredients:

- 1 cup brown basmati rice, rinsed and drained
- 1 cup dried green lentils, rinsed and drained
- 4 cups vegetable broth
- 1 tbsp. olive oil
- 1 onion, chopped
- 2 garlic cloves, minced
- 2 carrots, chopped
- 2 celery stalks, chopped
- 1 tsp ground cumin
- 1/2 tsp turmeric
- Salt and pepper
- Chopped fresh parsley, for garnish

Instructions:

1. In a large pot, heat olive oil over medium heat.
2. Add the chopped onion and garlic and cook until they start to soften, about 5 minutes.
3. Add the chopped carrot and celery and cook for another 5 minutes until they are slightly tender.
4. Stir in the ground cumin and turmeric and cook for an additional minute.
5. Add the rinsed and drained brown basmati rice, lentils, and vegetable broth to the pot.
6. Bring to a boil over high heat, cover and reduce heat to low and cook for 40-45 minutes or until lentils and rice are tender.
7. Season with salt and pepper, and serve hot garnished with chopped fresh parsley.

Nutritional Values per Person: Calories: 293 Fat: 5g Carbohydrates: 53g Fiber: 16g Protein: 13g

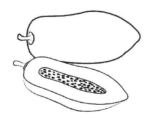

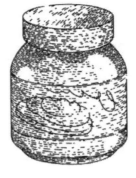

61. Whole Wheat Spaghetti with Broccoli Sauce

Difficulty: Easy   **Preparation Time:** 12 minutes

Cooking Time: 22 minutes   **Serving:** 4

Ingredients:

- 1 pound whole wheat spaghetti
- 2 tbsps. olive oil
- 1 onion, chopped
- 3 garlic cloves, minced
- 1 head of broccoli, chopped
- 2 cups vegetable broth
- Salt and pepper to taste
- Grated parmesan cheese, for garnish (optional)

Instructions:

1. Cook the whole wheat spaghetti according to package instructions and set aside.
2. Heat the oil in a pan over medium heat.
3. Add the minced garlic and onion and cook until soft and fragrant, about 6 minutes.
4. Add the chopped broccoli and vegetable broth to the pan and bring to a boil.
5. Reduce heat to medium and simmer until the broccoli is tender and the liquid has reduced, about 10-15 minutes.
6. Use a blender and make the mixture smooth and creamy.
7. Return the pureed broccoli sauce to the pan and season with pepper and salt to taste.
8. Add the cooked whole wheat spaghetti to the pan with the sauce and toss to coat evenly.
9. Serve hot with grated parmesan cheese, if desired.

Nutritional Values per Person: Calories: 400 Fat: 8g Carbohydrates: 70g Fiber: 12g Protein: 16g

62. Whole Wheat Pasta with Tuna and Tomato Sauce

Difficulty: Easy   **Preparation Time:** 10 minutes

Cooking Time: 20 minutes   **Serving:** 4

Ingredients:

- 1 pound whole wheat pasta
- 2 tbsps. olive oil
- 1 onion, chopped
- 3 garlic cloves, minced
- 1 can of tuna, drained
- 1 can of diced tomatoes
- Salt and pepper to taste
- Fresh parsley, chopped, for garnish (optional)

Instructions:

1. Cook the whole wheat pasta according to package instructions.
2. Heat the oil in a skillet over medium heat.
3. Add the chopped garlic and onion and cook until they are soft and fragrant about 6 minutes.
4. Add the drained tuna and diced tomatoes to the pan and bring to a simmer.
5. Reduce heat to medium-low and continue to cook until the sauce has thickened, about 10-15 minutes.
6. Season with salt and pepper.
7. Serve the tuna and tomato sauce over the cooked whole wheat pasta.
8. Garnish with fresh parsley, if desired.

Nutritional Values per Person: Calories: 375 Fat: 9g Carbohydrates: 55g Fiber: 10g Protein: 23g

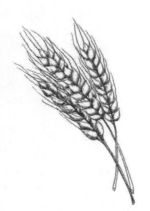

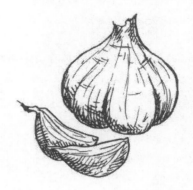

63. Whole Wheat Linguine with Lemon and Garlic Sauce

Difficulty: Easy   **Preparation Time:** 10 minutes

Cooking Time: 15 minutes   **Serving:** 4

Ingredients:

- 1 pound whole wheat linguine
- 3 garlic cloves, minced
- 2 lemons, juiced and zested
- 1/4 cup olive oil
- Salt and pepper
- Fresh parsley, chopped, for garnish (optional)

Instructions:

1. Cook the whole wheat linguine according to package instructions and set aside.

2. In a small bowl, mix together the minced garlic, lemon zest, lemon juice, olive oil, pepper and salt.

3. In a large pan, heat the lemon-garlic sauce over medium heat until it starts to simmer.

4. Add the cooked whole wheat linguine to the pan and toss to coat evenly with the sauce.

5. Let the linguine and sauce cook together for 1-2 minutes, stirring occasionally.

6. Season with additional salt and pepper, if needed.

7. Serve the linguine, garnishing with parsley.

Nutritional Values per Person: Calories: 395 Fat: 10g Carbohydrates: 64g Fiber: 10g Protein: 14g

64. Whole Wheat Spaghetti with Spinach and Mushroom Sauce

Difficulty: Easy   **Preparation Time:** 12 minutes

Cooking Time: 22 minutes   **Serving:** 4

Ingredients:

- 1 pound whole wheat spaghetti2 tbsps. olive oil
- 3 garlic cloves, minced
- 8 ounces mushrooms, sliced
- 4 cups fresh spinach, chopped
- 1/2 cup vegetable broth
- Salt and pepper to taste
- Fresh grated Parmesan cheese for topping (optional)

Instructions:

1. Cook the whole wheat spaghetti according to package instructions and set aside.
2. Heat the oil in a skillet over medium heat.
3. Add the minced garlic to the pan and cook for 2-3 minutes until fragrant.
4. Add the sliced mushrooms to the pan and sauté for 5-7 minutes until they are browned and tender.
5. Add the chopped spinach to the pan and stir until it wilts down.
6. Pour in the vegetable broth and stir to combine with the vegetables.
7. Season with salt and pepper.
9. Let the sauce simmer for 5-10 minutes to allow the flavors to blend together.
10. Serve the spaghetti with the spinach and mushroom sauce on top.
11. Top with fresh grated Parmesan cheese, if desired.

Nutritional Values per Person: Calories: 365 Fat: 7g Carbohydrates: 64g Fiber: 11g Protein: 14g

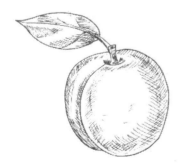

65. Whole Wheat Fettuccine with Shrimp and Tomato Sauce

Difficulty: Medium   **Preparation Time:** 15 minutes

Cooking Time: 25 minutes   **Serving:** 4

Ingredients:

- 1 pound whole wheat fettuccine
- 1 pound shrimp, peeled and deveined2 tbsps. olive oil
- 1 onion, chopped
- 2 garlic cloves, minced
- 1 tbsp. tomato paste
- 1 can (28 ounces) crushed tomatoes
- 1/2 tsp dried oregano
- Salt and pepper to taste
- Fresh basil leaves for topping (optional)

Instructions:

1. Cook the whole wheat fettuccine according to package instructions and set aside.
2. Heat the oil in a skillet over medium heat.
3. Add the chopped onion to the pan and sauté for 2-3 minutes until translucent.
4. Add the minced garlic to the pan and sauté for 2-3 minutes until fragrant.
5. Add the tomato paste to the pan and stir to combine with the onions and garlic.
6. Pour in the crushed tomatoes and stir to combine.
7. Add the dried oregano to the pan and season with salt and pepper to taste.
8. Let the sauce simmer over low heat for 10-15 minutes to allow the flavors to meld together.
9. Add the shrimp to the pan and cook for 4-5 minutes, stirring occasionally, until they are pink and cooked through.
10. Serve the whole wheat fettuccine with the shrimp and tomato sauce on top.
11. Top with fresh basil leaves, if desired.

Nutritional Values per Person: Calories: 400 Fat: 8g Carbohydrates: 59g Fiber: 11g Protein: 27g

66. Whole Wheat Penne with Chicken and Broccoli

Difficulty: Easy   **Preparation Time:** 15 minutes

Cooking Time: 30 minutes   **Serving:** 4

Ingredients:

- 1 pound boneless, skinless chicken breasts, cut into small pieces
- 1 pound whole wheat penne pasta
- 2 tbsps. olive oil
- 2 garlic cloves, minced
- 1 head of broccoli, cut into small florets
- 1/2 cup low-sodium chicken broth
- 1/4 cup grated parmesan cheese
- Salt and pepper to taste

Instructions:

1. Cook the whole wheat penne pasta according to package instructions.
2. Heat the oil in a skillet over medium heat.
3. Add the minced garlic to the pan and sauté for 1-2 minutes until fragrant.
4. Add the chicken breast pieces to the pan and cook for 5-7 minutes, stirring occasionally, until browned on all sides.
5. Add the broccoli florets to the pan and cook for an additional 3-4 minutes until slightly tender.
6. Pour in the low-sodium chicken broth and cook for 2-3 minutes until the broth has reduced slightly.
7. Add the cooked whole wheat penne pasta to the pan and stir to combine with the chicken and broccoli.
8. Add the grated parmesan cheese to the pan and stir to combine.
9. Season with salt and pepper.
10. Let the mixture simmer for an additional 2-3 minutes until the cheese has melted and the sauce has thickened.
11. Serve hot and enjoy!

Nutritional Values per Person: Calories: 460 Fat: 9g Carbohydrates: 59g Fiber: 11g Protein: 38g

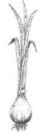

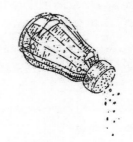

67. Farro Salad with Roasted Vegetables

Difficulty: Easy   **Preparation Time:** 15 minutes

Cooking Time: 30 minutes   **Serving:** 4

Ingredients:

- 1 cup uncooked farro
- 4 cups mixed vegetables (such as zucchini, bell peppers, and onions), chopped into small pieces
- 2 tbsps. olive oil
- 1/2 tsp salt
- 1/4 tsp black pepper
- 1/4 cup chopped fresh parsley
- 2 tbsps. red wine vinegar
- 2 tbsps. lemon juice
- 1 clove garlic, minced

Instructions:

1. Turn on the oven and bring it to 400°F.
2. Cook the spelled according to the instructions on the package and let it cool.
3. In a large bowl, toss the chopped vegetables in olive oil, salt, and pepper until evenly coated.
4. Spread the vegetables in a single layer on a baking sheet and place in the oven for 25-30 minutes, until golden brown and tender.
5. While the vegetables are roasting, prepare the dressing. In a bowl, whisk together the chopped parsley, red wine vinegar, lemon juice, and minced garlic.
6. Once the vegetables are done roasting, remove them from the oven and let them cool.
7. In a large bowl, combine the cooked farro and roasted vegetables.
8. Mix the dressing by pouring it over the spelled and vegetables.
9. Serve the farro salad immediately, or refrigerate until ready to serve.

Nutritional Values per Person: Calories: 340 Fat: 8g Carbohydrates: 60g Fiber: 13g Protein: 10g

68. Brown Rice and Lentil Bowl

Difficulty: Easy   **Preparation Time:** 12 minutes
Cooking Time: 40 minutes   **Serving:** 4
Ingredients:

- 1 cup brown rice
- 1 cup green lentils
- 4 cups vegetable broth
- 1 tbsp. olive oil
- 1/2 tsp salt
- 1/4 tsp black pepper
- 2 cups mixed vegetables (such as carrots, bell peppers, and broccoli), chopped into small pieces
- 1 avocado, sliced
- 1/4 cup chopped fresh cilantro
- 2 tbsps. lemon juice

Instructions:

1. Rinse the brown rice and lentils in a fine mesh strainer.
2. In a pot, bring the vegetable broth to a boil. Add the rice and lentils and stir to combine.
3. Cover with a lid and reduce the heat to low, and simmer for 35-40 minutes, until the rice and lentils are tender and the liquid is almost completely absorbed.
4. While the rice and lentils are cooking, heat the oil in a large skillet over medium heat.
5. Add the mixed vegetables, black pepper and salt to the skillet and cook for 5-7 minutes, until the vegetables are tender-crisp.
6. Once the rice and lentils are done cooking, remove from heat and let them sit covered for an additional 5 minutes.
7. Fluff the rice and lentils with a fork and divide among 4 bowls.
8. Top each bowl with the cooked vegetables, sliced avocado, and chopped cilantro.
9. Drizzle lemon juice over each bowl and serve.

Nutritional Values per Person: Calories: 420 Fat: 12g Carbohydrates: 64g Fiber: 18g Protein: 17g

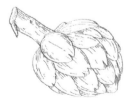

69. Quinoa and Veggie Stuffed Peppers

Difficulty: Moderate   **Preparation Time:** 20 minutes
Cooking Time: 45 minutes   **Serving:** 6
Ingredients:

- 6 large bell peppers, tops cut off and seeded
- 1 cup quinoa
- 2 cups vegetable broth
- 1 tbsp. olive oil
- 1 small onion, diced
- 2 garlic cloves, minced
- 1 tsp ground cumin
- 1/2 tsp paprika
- 1/2 tsp dried oregano
- 1/2 tsp salt
- 1/4 tsp black pepper
- 1 can (15 oz.) black beans, rinsed and drained
- 1 can (14 oz.) diced tomatoes, drained
- 1 cup frozen corn kernels
- 2 tbsps. chopped fresh cilantro
- 1/2 cup shredded cheddar cheese

Instructions:

1. Turn on the oven and bring it to 375°F.
2. In a medium saucepan, bring the quinoa and vegetable broth to a boil. Cover the pan and set the heat to low for 17-22 minutes until the liquid has been absorbed and the quinoa is tender.
3. While the quinoa is cooking, heat the olive oil in a large skillet over medium heat.
4. Sauté the onion and garlic until soft and translucent.
5. Add the cumin, paprika, oregano, salt, and black pepper to the skillet and cook for an additional minute.
6. Add the black beans, diced tomatoes, and corn to the skillet and stir to combine.
7. Stir in the cooked quinoa and chopped cilantro.
8. Stuff each bell pepper with the quinoa mixture and place in a baking dish.
9. Coat each pepper with grated cheese.
10. Line the pan with parchment paper and bake for 30 to 35 minutes, until the peppers are tender and the cheese has melted.
11. Remove the pan from the oven and let it cool for a few minutes. Have a good meal!

Nutritional Values per Person: Calories: 253 Fat: 8g Carbohydrates: 36g Fiber: 9g Protein: 12g

70. Barley and Vegetable Soup

Difficulty: Easy   **Preparation Time:** 10 minutes

Cooking Time: 45 minutes   **Serving:** 6

Ingredients:

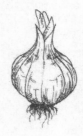

- 1 cup pearled barley
- 2 tbsps. olive oil
- 1 onion, chopped
- 2 garlic cloves, minced
- 3 carrots, chopped
- 3 celery stalks, chopped
- 6 cups vegetable broth
- 1 can (14 oz.) diced tomatoes, undrained
- 1 tsp dried basil
- 1 tsp dried oregano
- Salt and pepper to taste
- 2 cups chopped kale

Instructions:

1. Rinse the barley under running water and let it drain.
2. In a saucepan, heat the oil over medium heat.
3. Add the garlic and onion to the pot and sauté for 6 minutes.
4. Add the carrots and celery to the pot and continue to sauté for 6 minutes.
5. Add the vegetable broth, diced tomatoes, barley, basil, oregano, pepper and salt to the pot.
6. Bring the soup to a boil and turn the heat down to a simmer, cover the pot, and simmer for 30-35 minutes or until the barley is tender.
7. Stir in the chopped kale and cook for an additional 5 minutes, until the kale is wilted.

Nutritional Values per Person: Calories: 223 Fat: 6g Carbohydrates: 39g Fiber: 9g Protein: 8g

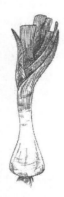

71. Millet and Chickpea Bowl

Difficulty: Easy   **Preparation Time:** 15 minutes

Cooking Time: 25 minutes   **Serving:** 4

Ingredients:

- 1 cup millet
- 2 cups vegetable broth
- 1 can (15 oz.) chickpeas, drained and rinsed
- 1 red bell pepper, sliced
- 1 yellow bell pepper, sliced
- 1 onion, sliced
- 2 tbsps. olive oil
- 2 garlic cloves, minced
- 1 tsp smoked paprika
- 1 tsp ground cumin
- Salt and pepper to taste
- 2 cups baby spinach leaves
- Juice of 1 lemon

Instructions:

1. Rinse the millet under cold running water and drain.
2. In a medium-sized pot, bring the vegetable broth to a boil. Add the millet and put the flame to a minimum, cover the pot, and simmer for 22-26 minutes or until the millet is tender.
3. While the millet is cooking, heat the oil in a large skillet over medium heat.
4. Add the bell peppers and onion to the skillet and sauté until the onion is soft and translucent and the peppers are slightly caramelized.
5. Add the garlic, smoked paprika, cumin, pepper, and salt to the skillet, and stir until fragrant.
6. Add the chickpeas to the skillet and stir to combine, cooking until they are heated through.
7. Once the millet is cooked, add the baby spinach leaves to the pot and stir until wilted.
8. Divide the millet and chickpea mixture between four bowls, and top each bowl with a squeeze of lemon juice.

Nutritional Values per Person: Calories: 326 Fat: 10g Carbohydrates: 49g Fiber: 10g Protein: 12g

72. Wheat Berry and Broccoli Salad

Difficulty: Easy **Preparation Time:** 22 minutes

Cooking Time: 45 minutes **Serving:** 4

Ingredients:

- 1 cup wheat berries
- 3 cups water
- 1 head of broccoli, cut into small florets
- 1 red onion, chopped
- 1 carrot, peeled and grated
- 1/2 cup dried cranberries
- 1/2 cup almonds, chopped
- 1/4 cup fresh parsley, chopped
- 1/4 cup fresh mint, chopped
- 3 tbsps. olive oil
- 2 tbsps. apple cider vinegar
- 1 tbsp. honey
- Salt and pepper

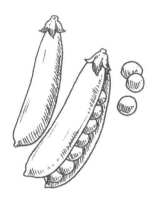

Instructions:

1. Rinse the wheat grains under water and drain them.
2. In a medium-sized pot, bring the water to a boil. Add the wheat kernels, cover pot and reduce heat to low, simmer 45 minutes or until wheat kernels are tender but still chewy.
3. While the wheat berries are cooking, steam the broccoli florets for 4-5 minutes until they are tender but still crisp.
4. In a large bowl, combine the cooked wheat berries, steamed broccoli, chopped red onion, grated carrot, dried cranberries, chopped almonds, parsley, and mint.
5. In a small mixing bowl, whisk together the olive oil, apple cider vinegar, honey, salt, and pepper.
6. Pour the dressing over the salad and toss until everything is coated.
7. Serve the salad chilled.

Nutritional Values per Person: Calories: 366 Fat: 17g Carbohydrates: 49g Fiber: 13g Protein: 10g

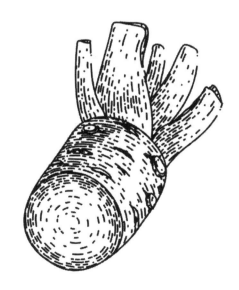

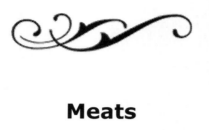

Meats

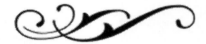

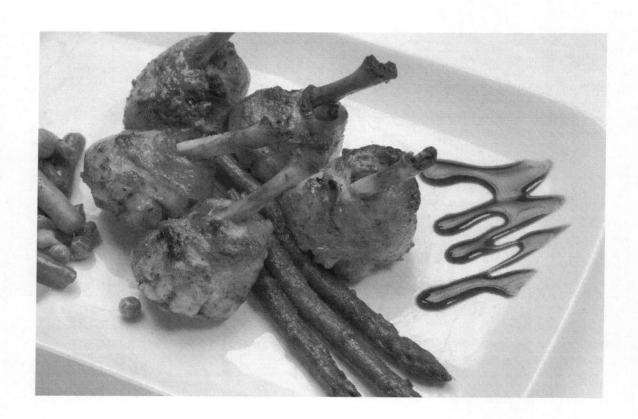

73. Grilled Chicken with Vegetables

Difficulty: Easy   **Preparation Time:** 22 minutes

Cooking Time: 20 minutes   **Serving:** 4

Ingredients:

- 4 boneless, skinless chicken breasts
- 2 tbsps. olive oil
- 1 tbsp. dried oregano
- 1 tsp garlic powder
- Salt and pepper to taste
- 1 red bell pepper, sliced
- 1 green bell pepper, sliced
- 1 zucchini, sliced
- 1 yellow squash, sliced
- 1 red onion, sliced
- 2 tbsps. balsamic vinegar
- 2 tbsps. chopped fresh parsley

Instructions:

1. Light the heat on the grill and heat it over medium-high heat.
2. In a bowl, mix together the oil, garlic powder, dried oregano, pepper and salt.
3. Brush the chicken breasts with the olive oil mixture.
4. Grill the chicken until cooked through for 6 to 8 minutes per side.
5. While the chicken is cooking, place the sliced vegetables in a large bowl. Toss them with the balsamic vinegar and season with salt and pepper to taste.
6. When the chicken is cooked, turn off the grill and remove it, leaving it to rest for about 5 minutes.
7. While chicken rests, grill vegetables 2 to 3 minutes per side or until lightly charred.
8. Slice the chicken and serve it with the vegetables. Garnish with chopped fresh parsley.

Nutritional Values per Person: Calories: 295 Fat: 11g Carbohydrates: 10g Fiber: 3g Protein: 37g

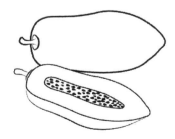

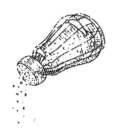

74. Turkey Meatballs

Difficulty: Easy   **Preparation Time:** 15 minutes

Cooking Time: 20 minutes

Serving: 4

Ingredients:

- 1 lb. ground turkey
- 1/2 cup whole wheat breadcrumbs
- 1/4 cup finely chopped onion
- 2 cloves garlic, minced
- 1 tsp dried oregano
- Salt and pepper to taste
- 1 egg, lightly beaten
- 1 tbsp. olive oil
- 1 can (14.5 oz.) diced tomatoes, no salt added
- 1/4 cup chopped fresh basil
- 1/4 cup grated parmesan cheese

Instructions:

1. Turn on the oven and bring it to 375°F.
2. In a large bowl, mix together the ground turkey, whole wheat breadcrumbs, chopped onion, minced garlic, dried oregano, salt, pepper, and beaten egg until well combined.
3. Scoop out small portions of the meat mixture and form into 1-inch meatballs.
4. In a pan, heat the oil over high heat. Add the meatballs and cook them until they are golden brown.
5. Transfer the meatballs to a baking dish, leaving any excess oil in the skillet.
6. In the same skillet, add the diced tomatoes and fresh basil. Cook for 3-4 minutes or until heated through.
7. Pour the tomato mixture over the meatballs in the baking dish.
8. Sprinkle the grated parmesan cheese over the top of the meatballs.
9. Bake in the preheated oven for 22 minutes or until the meatballs are cooked through.

Nutritional Values per Person: Calories: 250 Fat: 11g Carbohydrates: 13g Fiber: 3g Protein: 23g

75. Grilled Lamb with Vegetables

Difficulty: Intermediate   **Preparation Time:** 22 minutes + marinating time

Cooking Time: 16 minutes   **Serving:** 4

Ingredients:

- 1 lb. boneless leg of lamb, trimmed of fat and cut into 1-inch cubes
- 1 red bell pepper, seeded and cut into 1-inch pieces
- 1 yellow bell pepper, seeded and cut into 1-inch pieces
- 1 zucchini, sliced into 1/4-inch rounds
- 1 yellow squash, sliced into 1/4-inch rounds
- 1 red onion, cut into 1-inch pieces
- 2 cloves garlic, minced
- 2 tbsps. extra-virgin olive oil
- 2 tbsps. fresh lemon juice
- 1 tsp dried oregano
- Salt and pepper to taste
- Skewers

Instructions:

1. In a large bowl, mix together the lamb cubes, bell peppers, zucchini, yellow squash, red onion, minced garlic, olive oil, lemon juice, dried oregano, salt, and pepper. Cover and marinate in the refrigerator for at least 2 hours or overnight.
2. Preheat grill to medium-high heat
3. Thread the lamb and vegetables onto skewers, alternating the different ingredients.
4. Grill the skewers for about 10-15 minutes or until desired doneness.
5. Serve immediately.

Nutritional Values per Person: Calories: 300 Fat: 15g Carbohydrates: 10g Fiber: 3g Protein: 30g

76. Baked Chicken Sausages

Difficulty: Easy   **Preparation Time:** 12 minutes

Cooking Time: 30 minutes   **Serving:** 4

Ingredients:

- 4 chicken sausages
- 1 red bell pepper, sliced
- 1 yellow bell pepper, sliced
- 1 red onion, sliced
- 2 cloves garlic, minced
- 2 tbsps. extra-virgin olive oil
- Salt and pepper to taste
- Fresh parsley for garnish

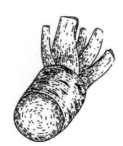

Instructions:

1. Turn on the oven and bring it to 400°F (200°C).
2. In a bowl, mix together the sliced bell peppers, sliced red onion, minced garlic, extra-virgin olive oil, salt, and pepper.
3. Place the chicken sausages on a baking dish, and surround them with the vegetable mixture.
4. Bake for 25-30 minutes, or until sausages and vegetables are cooked through.
5. Garnish with fresh parsley and serve immediately.

Nutritional Values per Person: Calories: 250 Fat: 15g Carbohydrates: 10g Fiber: 2g Protein: 20g

77. Chicken and Broccoli Air-Fry

Difficulty: Easy   **Preparation Time:** 12 minutes

Cooking Time: 15 minutes   **Serving:** 4

Ingredients:

- 1 pound boneless, skinless chicken breasts, cut into bite-sized pieces
- 2 cups broccoli florets
- 2 tbsps. olive oil
- 1 tsp garlic powder
- 1 tsp paprika
- 1 tsp dried oregano
- Salt and pepper

Instructions:

1. Preheat the air fryer to 375°F (190°C).
2. In a large bowl, mix together the chicken pieces, broccoli florets, oil, garlic powder, paprika, dried oregano, pepper, and salt.
3. Place the chicken and broccoli mixture into the air fryer basket.
4. Cook in the preheated air fryer for 13-16 minutes, or until the chicken is cooked through and the broccoli is crispy and tender.
5. Serve hot and enjoy!

Nutritional Values per Person: Calories: 250 Fat: 10g Carbohydrates: 10g Fiber: 3g Protein: 30g

78. Turkey and Vegetables Chili

Difficulty: Easy   **Preparation Time:** 16 minutes

Cooking Time: 30 minutes   **Serving:** 6

Ingredients:

- 1 pound lean ground turkey
- 1 tbsp. olive oil
- 1 large onion, chopped
- 2 bell peppers, chopped
- 3 garlic cloves, minced
- 2 tbsps. chili powder
- 1 tbsp. ground cumin
- 1 tsp smoked paprika
- 1 can (28 ounces) diced tomatoes, undrained
- 1 can (8 ounces) tomato sauce
- 1 can (15 ounces) kidney beans, drained and rinsed
- 1 can (15 ounces) corn, drained
- Salt and pepper to taste

Instructions:

1. In a pot or Dutch oven, heat oil over medium heat. Add ground turkey and cook until browned.
2. Add onion, bell pepper, and garlic to the pot, and cook until the vegetables are softened.
3. Add chili powder, ground cumin, and smoked paprika to the pot, and stir to combine.
4. Add diced tomatoes, tomato sauce, kidney beans, and corn to the pot, and stir to combine.
5. Bring the chili to a simmer, reduce heat, and cook for 20-25 minutes, or until the vegetables are tender and the flavors are well combined.
6. Season with salt and pepper.
7. Serve hot and enjoy!

Nutritional Values per Person: Calories: 290 Fat: 7g Carbohydrates: 35g Fiber: 7g Protein: 23g

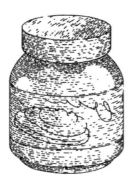

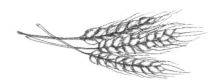

79. Turkey Meatballs with Zucchini Noodles

Difficulty: Easy   **Preparation Time:** 20 minutes

Cooking Time: 20 minutes   **Serving:** 4

Ingredients:

- 1 pound ground turkey
- 1 egg
- 1/4 cup breadcrumbs (use gluten-free if needed)
- 2 cloves garlic, minced
- 2 tbsps. fresh parsley, chopped
- Salt and pepper
- 2 large zucchinis, spiralizer
- 1 tbsp. olive oil
- 1/2 cup marinara sauce (use low-sugar if needed)
- Grated Parmesan cheese (optional)

Instructions:

1. Turn on the oven and bring it to 400 degrees F (200 degrees C).
2. In a large mixing bowl, combine ground turkey, egg, breadcrumbs, garlic, parsley, salt, and pepper.
3. Mix well and form into 12-16 meatballs.
4. Arrange the meatballs on a baking sheet and bake for about 18-20 minutes.
5. While the meatballs are baking, spiralizer zucchini into noodles using a spiralizer.
6. In a pan, heat the oil over medium heat.
7. Add zucchini noodles to the skillet and cook for 2-3 minutes, until slightly softened.
8. Add marinara sauce to the skillet and toss to coat the noodles.
9. Serve meatballs over zucchini noodles and top with grated Parmesan cheese, if desired.

Nutritional Values per Person: Calories: 291 Fat: 13g Carbohydrates: 12g Fiber: 3g Protein: 28g

80. Turkey Chili with Sweet Potatoes

Difficulty: Easy   **Preparation Time:** 20 minutes

Cooking Time: 45 minutes   **Serving:** 6

Ingredients:

- 1 pound ground turkey
- 1 onion, diced
- 4 cloves garlic, minced
- 1 tbsp. olive oil
- 1 tbsp. chili powder
- 1 tsp paprika
- 1 tsp cumin
- 1/2 tsp salt
- 1/4 tsp black pepper
- 2 large sweet potatoes, peeled and cubed
- 1 can (14 ounces) diced tomatoes
- 1 can (15 ounces) black beans, drained and rinsed
- 2 cups low-sodium chicken broth
- 1 tbsp. chopped fresh cilantro (optional)
- Sour cream and shredded cheddar cheese for serving (optional)

Instructions:

1. In a skillet, heat the oil over medium heat.
2. Add ground turkey, onion, and garlic to the pot.
3. Cook until turkey is browned and onions are softened, stirring occasionally.
4. Stir in chili powder, paprika, cumin, salt, and black pepper.
5. Add sweet potatoes, diced tomatoes, black beans, and chicken broth to the pot.
6. Bring to a boil and turn the heat down to low. Cook for 30-40 minutes until the potatoes are tender.
7. Stir in cilantro, if using.
8. Serve hot with a dollop of sour cream and shredded cheddar cheese, if desired.

Nutritional Values per Person: Calories: 275 Fat: 8g Carbohydrates: 32g Fiber: 8g Protein: 23g

81. Grilled Chicken with Roasted Beets

Difficulty: Easy   **Preparation Time:** 16 minutes

Cooking Time: 45 minutes   **Serving:** 4

Ingredients:

- 4 boneless, skinless chicken breasts
- 2 medium beets, peeled and diced
- 1 tbsp. olive oil
- 1 tbsp. balsamic vinegar
- 1/2 tsp dried rosemary
- 1/2 tsp salt
- 1/4 tsp black pepper
- 4 cups mixed greens
- 2 tbsps. chopped walnuts
- 1/4 cup crumbled goat cheese
- Balsamic vinaigrette for serving (optional)

Instructions:

1. Turn on the oven and bring it to 400°F.
2. In a large bowl, toss diced beets with olive oil, balsamic vinegar, rosemary, salt, and black pepper.
3. Arrange the beets in a layer on a baking sheet and roast for about 30-35 minutes or until tender.
4. In the meantime, heat a pan over high heat.
5. Season the chicken with pepper and salt.
6. Grill the chicken for 7-9 minutes per side, or until cooked through.
7. Let the chicken rest for 6 minutes, then slice it into strips.
8. To assemble the salad, divide mixed greens between four plates.
9. Top each plate with roasted beets, sliced chicken, chopped walnuts, and crumbled goat cheese.
10. Serve with balsamic vinaigrette, if desired.

Nutritional Values per Person: Calories: 306 Fat: 13g Carbohydrates: 9g Fiber: 3g Protein: 36g

44

82. Turkey and Spinach Burger

Difficulty: Easy   **Preparation Time:** 16 minutes

Cooking Time: 10 minutes   **Serving:** 4

Ingredients:

- 1 pound ground turkey
- 1/2 cup chopped spinach
- 1/4 cup chopped onion
- 1/4 cup bread crumbs
- 1 large egg
- 1 tbsp. Worcestershire sauce
- 1/2 tsp garlic powder
- 1/2 tsp salt
- 1/4 tsp black pepper
- 4 whole wheat buns
- Lettuce, tomato, and avocado, for topping (optional)

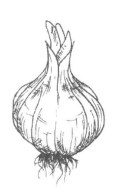

Instructions:

1. In a large bowl, mix together ground turkey, chopped spinach, onion, bread crumbs, egg, Worcestershire sauce, garlic powder, salt, and black pepper.
2. Divide the mixture into 4 parts and form hamburgers.
3. Heat a grill or grill pan over medium-high heat.
4. Cook the burger patties for 4-5 minutes per side, or until cooked through.
5. Toast the whole wheat buns on the grill for 1-2 minutes.
6. Serve the burgers on the buns with desired toppings (lettuce, tomato, and avocado, for example).

Nutritional Values per Person: Calories: 305 Fat: 12g Carbohydrates: 24g Fiber: 4g Protein: 28g

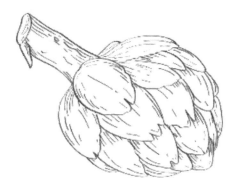

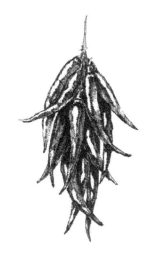

83. Turkey and Sweet Potato Burger

Difficulty: Easy   **Preparation Time:** 16 minutes

Cooking Time: 15 minutes   **Serving:** 4

Ingredients:

- 1 pound ground turkey
- 1 cup cooked and mashed sweet potato
- 1/4 cup chopped green onions
- 1/4 cup almond flour
- 1 large egg
- 1 tsp garlic powder
- 1/2 tsp cumin
- 1/2 tsp smoked paprika
- Salt and pepper to taste
- 4 whole wheat buns
- Lettuce, tomato, and red onion for topping (optional)

Instructions:

1. In a large bowl, mix together ground turkey, mashed sweet potato, green onions, almond flour, egg, garlic powder, cumin, smoked paprika, pepper, and salt.
2. Divide the mixture into 4 portions and shape them into hamburgers.
3. Heat a grill or grill pan over medium-high heat.
4. Cook the burger patties for 4-5 minutes per side, or until cooked through.
5. Toast the whole wheat buns on the grill for 1-2 minutes.
6. Assemble the burgers with desired toppings (lettuce, tomato, and red onion, for example).

Nutritional Values per Person: Calories: 310 Fat: 12g Carbohydrates: 25g Fiber: 5g Protein: 29g

84. Lamb Stew with Sweet Potato

Difficulty: Intermediate   **Preparation Time:** 20 minutes
Cooking Time: 2.5 hours   **Serving:** 4

Ingredients:

- 1 pound lamb meat, diced
- 1 large sweet potato, peeled and chopped
- 2 tbsps. olive oil
- 1 onion, diced
- 2 garlic cloves, minced
- 2 carrots, peeled and chopped
- 1 celery stalk, chopped
- 1 tbsp. tomato paste
- 2 cups beef broth
- 1 bay leaf
- 1/2 tsp thyme
- Salt and pepper to taste

Instructions:

1. In a pot, heat oil over medium heat. Add lamb meat and cook for 8-10 minutes or until browned. Remove the meat from the pot and set aside.
2. Add garlic and onion to the pot and cook for 2-3 minutes or until softened.
3. Add chopped sweet potato, carrots, and celery to the pot and cook for another 6 minutes.
4. Return the lamb meat to the pot and mix everything together.
5. Add tomato paste, beef broth, bay leaf, thyme, salt, and pepper to the pot. Stir everything together.
6. Cover the pot and simmer for 2 hours, stirring occasionally.
7. Remove the bay leaf before serving.

Nutritional Values per Person: Calories: 355 Fat: 17g Carbohydrates: 18g Fiber: 3g Protein: 31g

85. Grilled Turkey Cutlets

Difficulty: Easy   **Preparation Time:** 15 minutes
Cooking Time: 8 minutes   **Serving:** 4

Ingredients:

- 4 turkey cutlets
- 2 tbsps. olive oil
- 1 tsp dried rosemary
- Salt and pepper to taste

Instructions:

1. Preheat a grill pan over high heat.
2. Brush both sides of the turkey cutlets with olive oil and season with dried rosemary, salt, and pepper.

3. Place the turkey cutlets on the grill pan and cook for 4 minutes on each side or until fully cooked.
5. Remove from the heat and let rest for 2-3 minutes before serving.

Nutritional Values per Person: Calories: 150 Fat: 6g Carbohydrates: 0g Fiber: 0g Protein: 23g

86. Chicken and Lentil Stew

Difficulty: Intermediate   **Preparation Time:** 22 minutes
Cooking Time: 1 hour 30 minutes   **Serving:** 4

Ingredients:

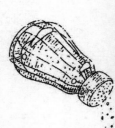

- 1 pound boneless chicken thighs, diced
- 1 cup dried lentils, rinsed and drained
- 2 tbsps. olive oil
- 1 onion, diced
- 2 garlic cloves, minced
- 2 carrots, peeled and chopped
- 1 celery stalk, chopped
- 1 tbsp. tomato paste
- 4 cups chicken broth
- 1 bay leaf
- 1/2 tsp thyme
- Salt and pepper to taste

Instructions:

1. In a pot, heat oil over medium heat. Add chicken and cook for 5-7 minutes or until browned. Remove the chicken from the pot and set aside.
2. Add garlic and onion to the pot and cook for 3-4 minutes or until softened.
3. Add chopped carrots and celery to the pot and cook for another 5 minutes.
4. Return the chicken to the pot and add lentils, tomato paste, chicken broth, bay leaf, thyme, salt, and pepper. Stir everything together.
5. Cover the pot and simmer for 1 hour, stirring occasionally.
6. Uncover the pot and continue to simmer for an additional 15-30 minutes or until the lentils are tender and the stew has thickened.
7. Remove the bay leaf before serving.

Nutritional Values per Person: Calories: 365 Fat: 13g Carbohydrates: 26g Fiber: 11g Protein: 37g

87. Turkey and Butternut Squash Stew

Difficulty: Intermediate   **Preparation Time:** 20 minutes
Cooking Time: 45 minutes   **Serving:** 4

Ingredients:

- 1 pound ground turkey
- 1 tbsp. olive oil
- 1 onion, chopped
- 2 garlic cloves, minced
- 1 butternut squash, peeled and diced
- 4 cups chicken broth
- 1 tsp ground cumin
- 1 tsp dried thyme
- 1/4 tsp cayenne pepper
- Salt and pepper to taste
- Chopped fresh parsley for garnish (optional)

Instructions:

1. In a saucepan, heat the oil over medium heat. Add the garlic and onion cook until softened.
2. Add ground turkey to the pot and cook until browned, breaking it up into smaller pieces.
3. Add butternut squash to the pot, along with chicken broth, cumin, thyme, cayenne pepper, salt, and pepper. Bring to a simmer.
4. Cover and cook for 30 minutes, or until the butternut squash is tender.
5. Remove from heat and let sit for a few minutes. Serve hot, garnished with fresh parsley if desired.

Nutritional Values per Person: Calories: 285 Fat: 13g Carbohydrates: 19g Fiber: 3g Protein: 23g

88. Grilled Chicken Kebabs with Vegetables

Difficulty: Easy   **Preparation Time:** 15 minutes
Cooking Time: 15 minutes   **Serving:** 4

Ingredients:

- 1 pound boneless, skinless chicken breasts, cut into 1-inch pieces
- 1 red bell pepper, seeded and cut into 1-inch pieces
- 1 green bell pepper, seeded and cut into 1-inch pieces
- 1 yellow onion, peeled and cut into 1-inch pieces
- 1 zucchini, sliced into 1/4 inch rounds
- 1/4 cup olive oil
- 2 tbsps. lemon juice
- 1 tsp dried oregano
- 1/2 tsp paprika
- Salt and pepper

- Bamboo skewers, soaked in water for 30 minutes

Instructions:

1. Turn the burner on and heat the grill over medium heat.
2. In a bowl, whisk lemon juice, oil, oregano, paprika, pepper, and salt.
3. Thread chicken, peppers, onion, and zucchini onto skewers.
4. Brush the chicken and vegetables with the olive oil mixture.
5. Grill the skewers for about 10-15 minutes, or until the vegetables and chicken are cooked through.

Nutritional Values per Person: Calories: 295 Fat: 16g Carbohydrates: 12g Fiber: 3.5g Protein: 27g

89. Grilled Lamb Chops with Mint Sauce

Difficulty: Intermediate   **Preparation Time:** 10 minutes
Cooking Time: 15 minutes   **Serving:** 4

Ingredients:

- 8 lamb chops, trimmed of excess fat
- 1/2 tsp salt
- 1/2 tsp black pepper
- 2 cloves garlic, minced
- 2 tbsps extra-virgin olive oil
- 1/4 cup fresh mint leaves, chopped
- 1 tbsp. fresh lemon juice
- Bamboo skewers, soaked in water for 32 minutes

Instructions:

1. Turn on the stove and heat the grill to high heat.
2. Season lamb chops with black pepper and salt.
3. In a bowl, mix together garlic and olive oil, and then brush onto both sides of the lamb chops.
4. Thread the lamb chops onto skewers, and then grill for 5-6 minutes per side.
5. In a separate bowl, combine lemon juice and mint to make the mint sauce.
6. Serve lamb chops with mint sauce.

Nutritional Values per Person: Calories: 270 Fat: 19g Carbohydrates: 1g Fiber: 0g Protein: 23g

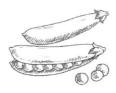

90. Grilled Turkey Burger with Avocado and Tomato

Difficulty: Easy   **Preparation Time:** 15 minutes

Cooking Time: 10 minutes   **Serving:** 4

Ingredients:

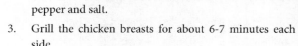

- 1 pound ground turkey
- 1/2 tsp garlic powder
- 1/2 tsp onion powder
- 1/2 tsp salt
- 1/4 tsp black pepper
- 4 whole wheat hamburger buns
- 1 avocado, sliced
- 1 tomato, sliced
- 4 leaves of lettuce

Instructions:

1. Place the grill on high heat.
2. In a medium bowl, mix ground turkey with onion powder, garlic powder, black pepper, and salt.
3. Form the turkey mixture into 4 equal sized patties.
4. Grill the turkey burgers for about 6 minutes.
5. While the burgers are cooking, slice the avocado, tomato, and lettuce.
6. To assemble the burgers, start with the bottom half of the bun, then add a lettuce leaf, followed by the turkey burger, sliced tomato, and avocado slices. Top the bun with the other half.

Nutritional Values per Person: Calories: 407 Fat: 18g Carbohydrates: 32g Fiber: 7g Protein: 32g

91. Grilled Chicken Breasts with Mango Salsa

Difficulty: Easy   **Preparation Time:** 16 minutes

Cooking Time: 16 minutes   **Serving:** 4

Ingredients:

- 4 boneless, skinless chicken breasts
- 1 tbsp. olive oil
- 1/2 tsp salt
- 1/4 tsp black pepper
- 1 mango, peeled and diced
- 1/2 red onion, diced
- 1/4 cup fresh cilantro, chopped
- 1 jalapeño pepper, seeded and minced
- 1 lime, juiced

Instructions:

1. Place the grill to heat over medium heat.

2. Rub the chicken breasts with oil and season with black pepper and salt.
3. Grill the chicken breasts for about 6-7 minutes each side.
4. While the chicken is cooking, prepare the mango salsa by combining diced mango, red onion, cilantro, jalapeño pepper, and lime juice in a small bowl.
5. Serve the grilled chicken breasts hot, topped with the mango salsa.

Nutritional Values per Person: Calories: 238 Fat: 5g Carbohydrates: 16g Fiber: 2g Protein: 34g

92. Grilled Turkey Skewers with Bell Peppers and Onions

Difficulty: Easy   **Preparation Time:** 25 minutes

Cooking Time: 16 minutes   **Serving:** 4

Ingredients:

- 1 pound turkey breast, cut into 1-inch cubes
- 1 red bell pepper, seeded and cut into 1-inch pieces
- 1 yellow bell pepper, seeded and cut into 1-inch pieces
- 1 onion, cut into 1-inch pieces
- 2 tbsps. olive oil
- 2 cloves garlic, minced
- 1/2 tsp dried oregano
- 1/2 tsp salt
- 1/4 tsp black pepper
- Juice of 1 lemon

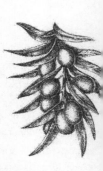

Instructions:

1. Place the grill on medium heat.
2. In a large bowl, combine turkey breast, bell peppers, onion, olive oil, oregano, garlic, black pepper, salt, and lemon juice. Toss to coat everything evenly.
3. Thread the turkey, bell peppers, and onion onto skewers, alternating between them.
4. Grill the skewers for about 12-14 minutes, turning often, until the vegetables are tender and the turkey is cooked through.
5. Serve hot, garnished with some extra lemon juice and fresh herbs, if desired.

Nutritional Values per Person: Calories: 242 Fat: 10g Carbohydrates: 10g Fiber: 2g Protein: 29g

93. Grilled Lamb Burger with Tzatziki Sauce

Difficulty: Intermediate   **Preparation Time:** 30 minutes

Cooking Time: 12 minutes   **Serving:** 4

Ingredients:

For the burgers:

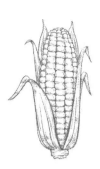

- 1 pound ground lamb
- 1/2 red onion, finely chopped
- 2 cloves garlic, minced
- 2 tbsps. chopped fresh parsley
- 1/2 tsp ground cumin
- 1/2 tsp paprika
- Salt and pepper, to taste
- 4 whole grain hamburger buns
- 4 lettuce leaves

For the tzatziki sauce:

- 1/2 cup plain Greek yogurt
- 1/4 cup grated cucumber
- 2 tbsps. chopped fresh dill
- 2 cloves garlic, minced
- 1/2 tsp lemon juice
- Salt and pepper, to taste

Instructions:

1. Place the grill over medium high heat.
2. In a large bowl, combine ground lamb, red onion, garlic, parsley, cumin, paprika, salt, and pepper. Mix well, making sure all ingredients are evenly distributed.
3. Take the compound and divide it into 4 and form the meatballs
4. Grill the patties for about 5-6 minutes on each side or until cooked to your liking.
5. While the burgers are cooking, prepare the tzatziki sauce. In a small bowl, combine, grated cucumber, Greek yogurt dill, lemon juice, garlic, salt, and pepper. Stir well to combine.
6. Toast the hamburger buns on the grill for a minute or two, until lightly charred.
7. To assemble the burgers, place a lettuce leaf on the bottom half of each bun, followed by a grilled lamb patty, and a generous dollop of tzatziki sauce. Top with the other half of the bun and serve hot.

Nutritional Values per Person: Calories: 404 Fat: 21g Carbohydrates: 25g Fiber: 5g Protein: 29g

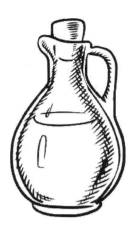

94. Grilled Lemon and Garlic Chicken Breasts

Difficulty: Easy   **Preparation Time:** 12 minutes

Cooking Time: 20 minutes   **Serving:** 4

Ingredients:

- 4 boneless, skinless chicken breasts
- 1/4 cup olive oil
- 1/4 cup lemon juice
- 2 garlic cloves, minced
- 1 tsp dried oregano
- Salt and pepper, to taste

Instructions:

1. Place the grill over medium-high heat
2. In a bowl, whisk together oil, garlic, lemon juice, salt, oregano, and pepper.
3. Place the chicken breasts in a shallow dish and pour the lemon-garlic marinade over them. Make sure the chicken is evenly coated.
4. Let the chicken marinate for 10-15 minutes while the grill heats up.
5. Place the chicken breasts on the grill and cook for about 8-10 minutes on each side or until the internal temperature reaches 165°F.
6. Turn off the heat, remove the chicken from the grill and let it rest for a few minutes.
7. Slice it and serve it.

Nutritional Values per Person: Calories: 235 Fat: 11g Carbohydrates: 2g Fiber: 0g Protein: 31g

95. Grilled Rosemary Balsamic Chicken Skewers

Difficulty: Easy   **Preparation Time:** 16 minutes

Cooking Time: 12 minutes   **Serving:** 4

Ingredients:

- 4 boneless, skinless chicken breasts, cut into cubes
- 1/4 cup balsamic vinegar
- 2 tbsps. olive oil
- 2 cloves garlic, minced
- 1 tbsp. fresh rosemary, minced
- Salt and pepper, to taste
- Skewers, soaked in water for 30 minutes (if using wooden skewers)

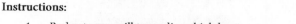

Instructions:

1. Put the grill on the stove and heat it over medium high heat.
2. In a small bowl, whisk together balsamic vinegar, garlic, oil, rosemary, pepper and salt.
3. Place the chicken cubes in a shallow dish and pour the balsamic marinade over them. Make sure the chicken is evenly coated.
4. Let the chicken marinate for 10-15 minutes while the grill heats up.
5. Thread the marinated chicken cubes onto skewers.
6. Place the chicken skewers on the grill and cook for about 5-6 minutes on each side or until the internal temperature reaches 165°F.
7. Remove the chicken skewers from the grill and let them rest for a few minutes before serving.

Nutritional Values per Person: Calories: 235 Fat: 10g Carbohydrates: 3g Fiber: 0g Protein: 32g

96. Grilled Lemon and Herb Turkey Burger

Difficulty: Easy   **Preparation Time:** 15 minutes

Cooking Time: 10-12 minutes   **Serving:** 4

Ingredients:

- 1 lb. ground turkey
- 1/4 cup bread crumbs
- 2 tbsps. chopped fresh parsley
- 2 tbsps. chopped fresh cilantro
- 1 tbsp. chopped fresh dill
- 1 tbsp. lemon zest
- 1 tbsp. lemon juice
- Salt and pepper, to taste
- 4 burger buns
- Optional toppings: lettuce, tomato, onion, avocado

Instructions:

1. Preheat your grill to medium-high heat.
2. In a large bowl, mix together the ground turkey, bread crumbs, parsley, cilantro, dill, lemon zest, lemon juice, salt, and pepper.
3. Divide the mixture into 4 equal parts and form them into patties.
4. Place the patties on the grill and cook for 5-6 minutes on each side, or until the internal temperature reaches 165°F.
5. Toast the burger buns on the grill, if desired.
6. Assemble the burgers with your favorite toppings.

Nutritional Values per Person: Calories: 250 Fat: 12g Carbohydrates: 19g Fiber: 2g Protein: 19g

97. Grilled Herb and Mustard Chicken Thighs

Difficulty: Easy   **Preparation Time:** 12 minutes

Cooking Time: 22-25 minutes   **Serving:** 4

Ingredients:

- 8 chicken thighs, bone-in, skin-on
- 2 tbsps. Dijon mustard
- 2 tbsps. olive oil
- 1 tbsp. chopped fresh rosemary
- 1 tbsp. chopped fresh thyme
- Salt and pepper
- Optional toppings: lemon wedges, chopped parsley

Instructions:

1. Put the grill on the fire and heat it to medium-high heat
2. In a bowl, mix together the Dijon mustard, olive oil, thyme, rosemary, pepper, and salt.
3. Brush the mixture evenly over the chicken thighs.
4. Place the chicken thighs on the grill, skin-side down, and cook for 10-12 minutes.
5. Flip the chicken and cook for another 10-12 minutes.
6. Remove the chicken from the grill and let it rest for a few minutes.
7. Optional: serve with lemon wedges and chopped parsley.

Nutritional Values per Person: Calories: 380 Fat: 28g Carbohydrates: 2g Fiber: 0g Protein: 29g

98. Mediterranean Herb Lamb Meatballs

Difficulty: Medium   **Preparation Time:** 20 minutes

Cooking Time: 22 minutes   **Serving:** 4

Ingredients:

- 1 pound ground lamb
- 1 large egg
- 1/2 cup breadcrumbs (or almond flour for a low-carb option)
- 1/4 cup chopped fresh parsley
- 1/4 cup chopped fresh mint
- 1/4 cup chopped fresh cilantro
- 2 garlic cloves, minced
- 1 tsp ground cumin
- 1/2 tsp paprika
- Salt and pepper, to taste
- 2 tbsps. olive oil

Instructions:

1. Turn on the oven and bring it to 375°F.
2. In a mixing bowl, combine the ground lamb, egg, breadcrumbs/almond flour, parsley, mint, cilantro, garlic, cumin, paprika, salt, and pepper.
3. Mix all the ingredients by kneading with your hands.
4. Form the mixture into meatballs about 1 1/2 inches in diameter.
5. In a pan suitable for the oven, heat the oil.
6. Add the meatballs to the skillet, spaced apart so they aren't touching.
7. Cook for 3-4 minutes per side, or until browned all over.
8. Place the pan in the oven and cook for 10-12 minutes.
9. Remove the skillet from the oven and let the meatballs rest for a few minutes before serving.

Nutritional Values per Person:

- Calories: 350
- Fat: 24g
- Carbohydrates: 9g (5g net carbs)
- Fiber: 4g
- Protein: 23g

99. Turkey Zucchini Meatballs

Difficulty: Easy   **Preparation Time:** 20 minutes

Cooking Time: 20 minutes   **Serving:** 4

Ingredients:

- 1 pound ground turkey
- 2 cups grated zucchini (about 2 medium zucchinis)
- 1/2 onion, finely chopped
- 2 garlic cloves, minced
- 1/4 cup chopped fresh parsley
- 1/4 cup chopped fresh basil
- 1/4 cup grated Parmesan cheese
- 1/2 cup breadcrumbs (or almond flour for a low-carb option)
- 1 large egg
- Salt and pepper, to taste
- 2 tbsps. olive oil

Instructions:

1. Turn on the oven and bring it to 400°F.
2. In a mixing bowl, combine the ground turkey, grated zucchini, onion, garlic, parsley, basil, Parmesan cheese, breadcrumbs/almond flour, egg, salt, and pepper.
3. Mix all the ingredients well by kneading them with your hands.
4. Form the mixture into meatballs about 1 1/2 inches in diameter.
5. In a pan suitable for the oven, heat the oil over high heat.
6. Add the meatballs to the skillet, spaced apart so they aren't touching.
7. Cook for 3-4 minutes per side, or until browned all over.
8. Transfer the skillet to the oven and bake for 10-12 minutes.
9. Remove the skillet from the oven and let the meatballs rest for a few minutes before serving.

Nutritional Values per Person: Calories: 320 Fat: 18g Carbohydrates: 11g (6g net carbs) Fiber: 5g Protein: 27g

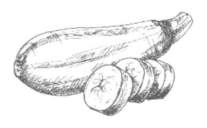

100. Ginger Lemon Chicken Meatballs

Difficulty: Easy   **Preparation Time:** 20 minutes

Cooking Time: 22 minutes   **Serving:** 4

Ingredients:

- 1 pound ground chicken
- 1/4 cup chopped green onions
- 3 garlic cloves, minced
- 1 tbsp. grated fresh ginger
- 2 tbsps. lemon juice
- 1/2 tsp salt
- 1/4 tsp black pepper
- 1/4 cup almond flour
- 1 large egg
- 2 tbsps. olive oil

Instructions:

1. Turn the oven to 400°F.
2. In a mixing bowl, combine the ground chicken, green onions, garlic, grated ginger, lemon juice, salt, black pepper, almond flour, and egg.
3. Mix with your hands until all ingredients are well combined.
4. Form the mixture into meatballs about 1 1/2 inches in diameter.
5. In a pan suitable for the oven, heat the oil over high heat.
6. Add the meatballs to the skillet, spaced apart so they aren't touching.
7. Cook for 3-4 minutes per side, or until browned all over.
8. Transfer the skillet to the oven and bake for 10-12 minutes.
9. Remove the skillet from the oven and let the meatballs rest for a few minutes before serving.

Nutritional Values per Person: Calories: 235 Fat: 16g Carbohydrates: 2g (1g net carbs) Fiber: 1g Protein: 20g

101. Turkey Fajitas with Peppers and Onions

Difficulty: Easy   **Preparation Time:** 12 minutes

Cooking Time: 15 minutes   **Serving:** 4

Ingredients:

- 1 pound ground turkey
- 2 bell peppers, sliced
- 1 onion, sliced
- 1 tbsp. chili powder
- 1/2 tsp cumin
- 1/4 tsp garlic powder
- Salt and pepper to taste
- 1 tbsp. olive oil
- 8 small flour tortillas
- Lime wedges and chopped fresh cilantro, for garnish

Instructions:

1. In a large frying pan, heat the oil over high heat.
2. Add the sliced peppers and onions and cook until softened, about 6 minutes.
3. Add the ground turkey to the skillet and cook until browned and cooked through, about 10 minutes.
4. Season with chili powder, garlic powder, pepper, cumin, and salt.
5. Heat the flour tortillas in the microwave or oven until warmed through.
6. Divide the turkey and pepper mixture among the tortillas and serve with lime wedges and chopped cilantro.

Nutritional Values per Person: Calories: 401 Fat: 16g Carbohydrates: 35g (6g net carbs) Fiber: 4g Protein: 29g

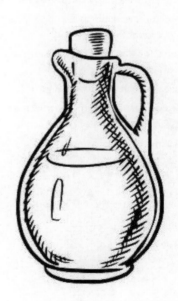

102. Baked Chicken Taco with Avocado and Tomatoes

Difficulty: Easy   **Preparation Time:** 15 minutes

Cooking Time: 22 minutes   **Serving:** 4

Ingredients:

- 4 small chicken breasts
- 6 corn tortillas
- 1 large avocado, diced
- 1 large tomato, diced
- 1/4 cup chopped fresh cilantro
- 1 tbsp. olive oil
- 1 tbsp. chili powder
- 1/2 tsp ground cumin
- 1/2 tsp garlic powder
- 1/2 tsp onion powder
- Salt and pepper to taste

Instructions:

1. Turn on the oven and bring it to 375°F.
2. In a small bowl, mix together the olive oil, chili powder, garlic powder, ground cumin, pepper, onion powder, and salt.
3. Brush the chicken breasts with the spice mixture and place them on a baking sheet.
4. Bake the chicken for 20 minutes, or until cooked through with no pink inside.
6. While the chicken is baking, heat the corn tortillas in the oven or microwave until warm.
7. Once the chicken is cooked, remove it from the oven and let it cool for a few minutes.
8. Cut the chicken into strips or small pieces.
9. Assemble the tacos by placing a couple of spoonfuls of chicken on top of each tortilla.
10. Top with diced avocado, diced tomato, and chopped cilantro.
11. Serve hot.

Nutritional Values per Person: Calories: 369 Fat: 18g Carbohydrates: 21g (6g net carbs) Fiber: 3g Protein: 33g

103. Turkey and Sugar Snap Pea Meatballs

Difficulty: Easy   **Preparation Time:** 22 minutes

Cooking Time: 30 minutes   **Serving:** 4

Ingredients:

- 1 pound ground turkey
- 1 cup sugar snap peas, finely chopped
- 1/2 cup almond flour
- 1 egg
- 1/4 cup chopped fresh parsley
- 1/4 tsp garlic powder
- Salt and pepper to taste
- 1 tbsp. olive oil

Instructions:

1. Turn on the oven and bring it to 375°F (190°C).
2. In a large mixing bowl, combine the ground turkey, chopped sugar snap peas, almond flour, egg, parsley, garlic powder, salt, and pepper.
3. Mix well until all ingredients are evenly combined.
4. Using a tbsp., scoop out the mixture and shape it into meatballs with your hands.
5. Arrange the meatballs on a baking sheet lined with parchment paper.
6. Brush the meatballs lightly with olive oil.
7. Bake for 26-30 minutes or until cooked through and golden brown.

Nutritional Values per Person: Calories: 247 Fat: 11g Carbohydrates: 7g (3g net carbs) Fiber: 4g Protein: 29g

104. Mediterranean Herb-Roasted Turkey Breast

Difficulty: Intermediate   **Preparation Time:** 20 minutes

Cooking Time: 1 hour and 35 minutes **Serving:** 8

Ingredients:

- 1 bone-in turkey breast (about 6 pounds)
- 1/4 cup olive oil
- 2 tbsps. fresh thyme leaves
- 2 tbsps. fresh rosemary leaves
- 1 tbsp. fresh sage leaves, chopped
- 1 tbsp. garlic powder
- Salt and pepper

Instructions:

1. Turn on the oven and bring it to 325°F (160°C).
2. Rinse the turkey breast and pat it dry with paper towels.
3. In a mixing bowl, whisk together the oil, thyme, rosemary, sage, garlic powder, pepper and salt.
4. Rub the herb mixture all over the turkey breast, making sure to get it under the skin.
5. Place the turkey breast on a roasting rack in a large roasting pan.
6. Roast for about 1 hour and 35 minutes.
7. Let the turkey breast rest for 10-15 minutes before slicing and serving.

Nutritional Values per Person: Calories: 358 Fat: 15g Carbohydrates: 2g (1g net carbs) Fiber: 1g Protein: 51g

105. Greek Yogurt Chicken Salad

Difficulty: Easy   **Preparation Time:** 16 minutes

Cooking Time: 16 minutes   **Serving:** 4

Ingredients:

- 2 chicken breasts, cooked and shredded
- 1/2 cup Greek yogurt
- 1/4 cup diced red onion
- 1/4 cup diced celery
- 1/4 cup chopped fresh parsley
- 1/4 cup chopped fresh dill
- 1 tbsp. lemon juice
- 1/2 tsp garlic powder
- Salt and pepper to taste

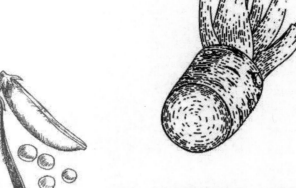

Instructions:

1. In a large mixing bowl, combine the shredded chicken, Greek yogurt, red onion, celery, parsley, dill, garlic powder, lemon juice, pepper, and salt.
2. Mix all the ingredients until they are well combined.
3. Chill the chicken salad in the refrigerator for at least 35 minutes before serving.
5. Serve the chicken salad on a bed of lettuce or in a sandwich.

Nutritional Values per Person: Calories: 192 Fat: 5g Carbohydrates: 6g (3g net carbs) Fiber: 3g Protein: 32g

106. Honey Mustard Chicken

Difficulty: Easy   **Preparation Time:** 10 minutes

Cooking Time: 20 minutes   **Serving:** 4

Ingredients:

- 4 boneless, skinless chicken breasts
- 1/4 cup Dijon mustard
- 2 tbsps. honey
- 2 tbsps. olive oil
- 1 garlic clove, minced
- Salt and pepper to taste

Instructions:

1. Turn on the oven and bring it to 375°F (190°C).
2. In a small mixing bowl, whisk together the Dijon mustard, honey, oil, garlic, pepper and salt.
3. Place the chicken breasts in a baking dish and pour the honey mustard mixture over them, making sure to coat them well.
4. Bake the chicken for 20-25 minutes.
5. Remove the chicken from the oven and let it rest for 6-7 minutes before serving.

Nutritional Values per Person: Calories: 250 Fat: 8g Carbohydrates: 11g (10g net carbs) Fiber: 1g Protein: 32g

107. Chinese BBQ Chicken Wings

Difficulty: Easy   **Preparation Time:** 12 minutes

Cooking Time: 22-25 minutes   **Serving:** 4

Ingredients:

- 2 lbs. chicken wings
- 1/4 cup low-sodium soy sauce
- 1/4 cup hoisin sauce
- 2 tbsps. honey
- 1 tbsp. grated fresh ginger
- 2 garlic cloves, minced
- Salt and pepper
- Scallions and sesame seeds for garnish

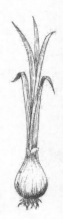

Instructions:

1. Turn on the oven and bring it to 425°F (218°C).
2. In a mixing bowl, whisk together the soy sauce, hoisin sauce, honey, ginger, garlic, pepper and salt.
3. Add the chicken wings to the mixing bowl and toss until they are coated in the marinade.
4. Line a baking sheet with aluminum foil and spray with cooking spray.
5. Place the chicken wings on the baking sheet and bake in the oven until crispy and cooked through, about 22-26 minutes.
6. Remove the chicken wings from the oven and let them sit for a few minutes before garnishing with scallions and sesame seeds.

Nutritional Values per Person: Calories: 278 Fat: 15g Carbohydrates: 12g (10g net carbs) Fiber: 1g Protein: 22g

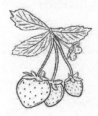

108. Chinese Five Spice Chicken

Difficulty: Easy **Preparation Time:** 12 minutes

Cooking Time: 20-25 minutes **Serving:** 4

Ingredients:

- 4 bone-in, skin-on chicken thighs
- 1 tsp Chinese five spice powder
- 2 tsps. low-sodium soy sauce
- 2 tsps. honey
- 2 garlic cloves, minced
- Salt and pepper to taste
- Scallions for garnish

Instructions:

1. Turn on the oven and bring it to 425°F (218°C).
2. In a small mixing bowl, whisk together the Chinese five spice powder, soy sauce, honey, garlic, salt, and pepper.
3. Place the chicken thighs on a baking sheet lined with aluminum foil.
4. Brush the chicken thighs generously with the spice mixture.
5. Bake the chicken thighs in the oven for 20-25 minutes.
6. Remove the chicken from the oven and let it rest for a few minutes before garnishing with scallions.

Nutritional Values per Person: Calories: 289 Fat: 17gCarbohydrates: 7g (6g net carbs) Fiber: 1gProtein: 26g

109. Thai Basil Chicken

Difficulty: Easy **Preparation Time:** 22 minutes

Cooking Time: 10 minutes **Serving:** 4

Ingredients:

- 1 lb. boneless, skinless chicken breast, cut into small pieces
- 2 tbsps. vegetable oil
- 4 garlic cloves, minced
- 2 fresh red chili peppers, sliced
- 1 red bell pepper, sliced
- 1 cup Thai basil leaves
- 2 tbsps. low-sodium soy sauce
- 2 tbsps. oyster sauce
- Salt and pepper
- Scallions for garnish

Instructions:

1. In a wok or large skillet, heat the vegetable oil over medium-high heat.
2. Add the minced garlic and stir-fry for 30 seconds or until fragrant.
3. Add the sliced chicken and stir-fry until it is browned and cooked through.
4. Add the sliced red bell pepper and fresh red chili peppers, and continue stir-frying for another minute.
5. Stir in the Thai basil leaves, soy sauce, oyster sauce, pepper, salt, and cook until the sauce has thickened and the basil leaves have wilted.
6. Remove the Thai basil chicken from the heat and serve hot garnished with scallions.

Nutritional Values per Person: Calories: 200 Fat: 10g Carbohydrates: 7g (4g net carbs) Fiber: 3g Protein: 19g

110. Green Curry Chicken

Difficulty: Moderate **Preparation Time:** 22 minutes

Cooking Time: 30 minutes **Serving:** 4

Ingredients:

- 1 lb. boneless, skinless chicken breast, cut into small pieces
- 2 tbsps. vegetable oil
- 1 can (14 oz.) coconut milk
- 2-3 tbsps. green curry paste
- 2 cups mixed vegetables (such as bell peppers, green beans, and zucchini), sliced
- 1 tbsp. fish sauce
- Juice of 1 lime
- Salt and pepper to taste
- Fresh cilantro for garnish

Instructions:

1. In a wok or large skillet, heat the vegetable oil over medium heat.
2. Add the green curry paste and stir-fry for 1-2 minutes.
3. Add the sliced chicken and stir-fry until it is browned and cooked through.
4. Add the mixed vegetables and continue stir-frying for 1-2 minutes.
5. Pour in the coconut milk, fish sauce, and lime juice, and bring the mixture to a simmer.
6. Lower the heat and let the curry simmer for 12-16 minutes.
7. Season the curry with pepper and salt to taste and serve hot, garnished with fresh cilantro.

Nutritional Values per Person: Calories: 375 Fat: 23g Carbohydrates: 14g (8g net carbs) Fiber: 6g Protein: 25g

111. Tom Kha Gai (Coconut Milk Soup with Chicken)

Difficulty: Easy   **Preparation Time:** 16 minutes

Cooking Time: 20 minutes   **Serving:** 4

Ingredients:

- 1 lb. boneless chicken breast, cut into bite-sized pieces
- 4 cups chicken broth
- 2 cans (14 oz. each) coconut milk
- 1 inch piece of fresh galangal or ginger, sliced
- 2 stalks lemongrass, bruised and chopped
- 4-5 kaffir lime leaves
- 2 tbsps. fish sauce
- 2 tbsps. lime juice
- 2 tbsps. brown sugar
- 1/2 cup mushrooms, sliced
- 1/2 cup cherry tomatoes
- Fresh cilantro leaves for garnish
- Red chili flakes (optional)

Instructions:

1. In a pot, bring the chicken broth to a boil over high heat.
2. Add the galangal or ginger, lemongrass, and kaffir lime leaves to the broth.
3. Reduce heat and simmer for 6 to 9 minutes to infuse the broth with the flavors.
4. Add the chicken to the pot and let it cook for 5-7 minutes or until fully cooked.
5. Add the coconut milk, fish sauce, lime juice, and brown sugar to the pot.
6. Add the sliced mushrooms and cherry tomatoes to the pot and let them cook for another 2-3 minutes.
7. Remove the pot from the heat and let it cool for 5-10 minutes before serving.
8. Garnish with fresh cilantro leaves and red chili flakes (optional).

Nutritional Values per Person: Calories: 327 Fat: 26g Carbohydrates: 8g (7g net carbs) Fiber: 1g Protein: 20g

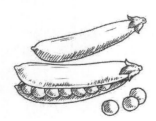

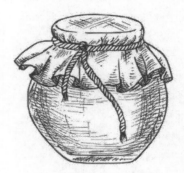

112. Lamb Meatballs with Mint

Difficulty: Easy   **Preparation Time:** 20 minutes

Cooking Time: 25 minutes   **Serving:** 4

Ingredients:

- 1 lb. ground lamb
- 1/2 cup breadcrumbs
- 1/4 cup fresh mint leaves, chopped
- 1/4 cup fresh parsley leaves, chopped
- 1 tbsp. ground cumin
- 1 tbsp. ground coriander
- 1 tsp smoked paprika
- 1/2 tsp salt
- 1/4 tsp black pepper
- 1 egg, beaten
- 1/4 cup olive oil

Instructions:

1. In a large bowl, mix together the ground lamb, breadcrumbs, chopped mint, chopped parsley, cumin, coriander, smoked paprika, salt, black pepper, and beaten egg until well combined.
2. Using your hands, shape the mixture into small meatballs.
3. In a large skillet heat the oil over medium-high heat.
4. Add the meatballs to the pan and cook for 4 to 5 minutes on each side.
5. Transfer the meatballs to a serving dish and garnish with extra fresh mint leaves.
6. Serve hot.

Nutritional Values per Person: Calories: 420 Fat: 32g Carbohydrates: 10g (2g net carbs) Fiber: 1g Protein: 23g

113. Larb Gai (Thai Minced Chicken Salad)

Difficulty: Easy **Preparation Time:** 22 minutes

Cooking Time: 10 minutes **Serving:** 4

Ingredients:

- 1 lb. ground chicken
- 2 tbsps. vegetable oil
- 1/4 cup lime juice
- 1 tbsp. fish sauce
- 1 tbsp. soy sauce
- 1 tbsp. honey
- 1/4 cup red onion, finely chopped
- 1/4 cup fresh mint leaves, chopped
- 1/4 cup fresh cilantro leaves, chopped
- 2 hot chili peppers, minced (optional)
- 1 head of lettuce, washed and leaves separated

Instructions:

1. In a large skillet, heat the oil over medium high heat.
2. Add the ground chicken to the skillet and cook for 5-6 minutes, stirring occasionally, or until browned and cooked through.
3. In a small bowl, whisk together the fish sauce, lime juice, soy sauce, and honey to make the dressing.
4. In a large mixing bowl, combine the cooked chicken, red onion, chopped mint leaves, chopped cilantro leaves, and minced chili peppers (if using).
5. Pour the dressing over the chicken mixture and toss to combine.
6. Arrange the lettuce leaves on a large serving platter.
7. Spoon the chicken salad mixture onto the lettuce leaves.
8. Garnish with extra mint and cilantro leaves, if desired.
9. Serve at room temperature.

Nutritional Values per Person: Calories: 240 Fat: 13g Carbohydrates: 11g (8g net carbs) Fiber: 3g Protein: 20g

114. Chicken Kofta

Difficulty: Moderate **Preparation Time:** 22 minutes

Cooking Time: 30 minutes **Serving:** 4

Ingredients:

- 1 lb. ground chicken
- 1/2 cup breadcrumbs
- 1 egg, lightly beaten
- 1 tsp ground cumin
- 1 tsp ground coriander
- 1 tsp garlic powder
- 1 tsp onion powder
- 1/2 tsp paprika
- 1/4 tsp cayenne pepper
- 1/4 cup fresh parsley, finely chopped
- Salt and pepper
- 2 tbsps. vegetable oil
- 1 onion, chopped
- 2 garlic cloves, minced
- 1 can (14.5 oz.) crushed tomatoes
- 1 cup chicken broth
- 1 tbsp. tomato paste
- Chopped fresh parsley or cilantro, for serving

Instructions:

1. Turn on the oven and bring it to 375°F (190°C).
2. In a mixing bowl, combine the ground chicken, breadcrumbs, egg, cumin, coriander, garlic powder, onion powder, paprika, cayenne pepper, fresh parsley, salt, and pepper.
3. Mix until all ingredients are well combined and form the mixture into small balls (about 1 1/2 inches in diameter).
4. Heat the vegetable oil in a skillet over medium heat.
5. Add the garlic and chopped onion and cook for 3-4 minutes.
6. Add the meatballs to the skillet and cook for 5-6 minutes, or until browned on all sides.
7. Transfer the patties to a baking sheet and bake in the oven for 15 to 20 minutes or until cooked through.
8. While the meatballs are baking, prepare the sauce. In the same skillet used to cook the meatballs, add the crushed tomatoes, chicken broth, and tomato paste.
9. Bring the sauce to a simmer and cook for 11-15 minutes, or until it has thickened.
10. Once the meatballs are done baking, add them to the skillet with the sauce and toss to coat.
11. Serve hot, garnished with chopped fresh parsley or cilantro, if desired.

Nutritional Values per Person: Calories: 320 Fat: 15g Carbohydrates: 19g (4g net carbs) Fiber: 3g Protein: 26g

Fish and Seafood

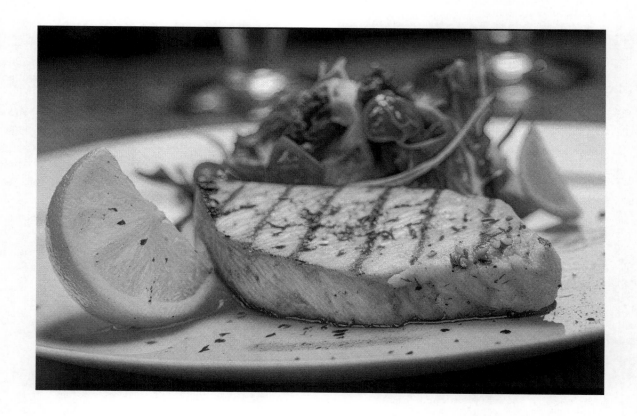

115. Pan-Seared Salmon with Sautéed Spinach

Difficulty: Easy   **Preparation Time:** 12 minutes

Cooking Time: 16 minutes   **Serving:** 2

Ingredients:

- 2 salmon fillets (6 oz. each), skin on
- Salt and pepper, to taste
- 1 tbsp. olive oil
- 2 garlic cloves, minced
- 1/2 tsp red pepper flakes (optional)
- 4 cups fresh spinach leaves, washed and trimmed
- 1 tbsp. lemon juice
- Lemon wedges, for serving

Instructions:

1. Rinse and pat dry the salmon fillets. Season both sides of the fillets with pepper and salt.
2. In a large nonstick skillet heat the oil over medium-high heat.
3. Add the salmon fillets to the skillet, skin-side down. Cook for 4-5 minutes.
4. Flip the salmon fillets and continue cooking for another 4-5 minutes.
5. Remove salmon from the skillet and place on a plate. Cover with foil to keep warm.
6. In the same skillet, add garlic and red pepper flakes (if using). Cook for 2 minutes or until fragrant.
7. Add the spinach leaves and cook for another 2-3 minutes until wilted.
8. Add lemon juice and season with salt and pepper to taste.
9. Serve the salmon fillets with sautéed spinach and lemon wedges.

Nutritional Values per Person: Calories: 320 Total Fat: 20g Saturated Fat: 3g Cholesterol: 80 mg Sodium: 400 mg Total Carbohydrate: 4g Dietary Fiber: 2g Sugar: 0g Protein: 31g

116. Cilantro Lime Salmon

Difficulty: Easy   **Preparation Time:** 16 minutes

Cooking Time: 12 minutes   **Serving:** 4

Ingredients:

- 4 salmon fillets (6 oz. each)
- Salt and pepper, to taste
- 2 tbsps. olive oil
- 1/4 cup fresh cilantro, chopped
- 2 garlic cloves, minced
- 2 tbsps. lime juice
- Lime wedges, for serving

Instructions:

1. Rinse and pat dry the salmon fillets. Season both sides of the fillets with pepper and salt.

2. In a large nonstick skillet heat the oil over medium-high heat.
3. Add the salmon fillets to the skillet, skin-side down. Cook for 4-5 minutes.
4. Flip the salmon fillets and continue cooking for another 4-5 minutes.
5. In a small bowl, mix together garlic, cilantro, and lime juice.
6. Brush the cilantro lime mixture over the salmon fillets in the skillet.
7. Cook for an additional 2 minutes until the sauce is heated through and lightly caramelized.
8. Serve the salmon fillets with lime wedges.

Nutritional Values per Person: Calories: 400 Total Fat: 26g Saturated Fat: 5g Cholesterol: 90mg Sodium: 150 mg Total Carbohydrate: 2g Dietary Fiber: 0g Sugar: 0g Protein: 33g

117. Salmon Cakes

Difficulty: Intermediate   **Preparation Time:** 20 minutes

Cooking Time: 20 minutes   **Serving:** 4

Ingredients:

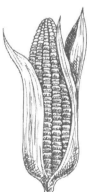

- 2 cans (14.75 oz. each) of wild caught salmon, drained and flaked
- 1/2 cup almond flour
- 2 eggs, beaten
- 2 tbsps. Dijon mustard
- 2 tbsps. chopped fresh parsley
- 1 tbsp. chopped fresh dill
- 1 tbsp. chopped fresh chives
- 2 cloves garlic, minced
- Salt and pepper
- 2 tbsps. olive oil
- Lemon wedges, for serving

Instructions:

1. In a large bowl, mix together the flaked salmon, almond flour, beaten eggs, Dijon mustard, chopped parsley, fresh dill, chives, minced garlic, salt, and pepper.
2. Stir the mixture until well combined and shape into patties.
3. Heat olive oil in a non-stick skillet over medium heat.
4. Add the salmon cakes to the skillet and cook for 4-5 minutes on each side.
5. Once cooked, remove salmon cakes from skillet and place on a plate lined with paper towels.
6. Serve with lemon wedges on the side.

Nutritional Values per Person: Calories: 350 Total Fat: 22g Saturated Fat: 3g Cholesterol: 140mg Sodium: 350mg Total Carbohydrate: 9g Dietary Fiber: 4g Sugar: 1g Protein: 33g

118. Salmon Air-Fry

Difficulty: Easy   **Preparation Time:** 6 minutes
Cooking Time: 10 minutes   **Serving:** 2

Ingredients:

- 2 salmon fillets (6-8 oz. each)
- 1 tbsp. olive oil
- 1 tsp smoked paprika
- 1/2 tsp garlic powder
- Salt and pepper
- Lemon wedges, for serving

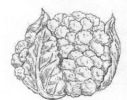

Instructions:

1. Turn on the air fryer and turn it on 400°F.
2. In a bowl, mix together the olive oil, smoked paprika, salt, garlic powder, and pepper.
3. Brush the mixture onto both sides of the salmon fillets.
4. Place the salmon fillets in the air fryer basket and cook for 8-10 minutes, or until the salmon is cooked through and tender.
5. Once cooked, remove the salmon from the air fryer basket and place on a plate.
6. Serve with lemon wedges on the side.

Nutritional Values per Person: Calories: 300 Total Fat: 16g Saturated Fat: 2.5g Cholesterol: 80 mg Sodium: 120mg Total Carbohydrate: 1g Dietary Fiber: 0g Sugar: 0g Protein: 35g

119. Baked Salmon with Asparagus

Difficulty: Easy   **Preparation Time:** 12 minutes
Cooking Time: 16-20 minutes   **Serving:** 4

Ingredients:

- 4 salmon fillets (6 oz. each)
- 1 bunch of asparagus, trimmed
- 2 tbsps. olive oil
- Salt and pepper, to taste
- 2 garlic cloves, minced
- 1 lemon, sliced
- Fresh parsley, chopped, for garnish

Instructions:

1. Turn on the oven and bring it to 400°F.
2. Line a baking sheet or dish with parchment paper.
3. Place the salmon fillets and asparagus on the baking sheet.
4. Drizzle the oil over the salmon and asparagus, and season with salt and pepper to taste.
5. Add the minced garlic to the salmon and asparagus.
6. Place lemon slices on top of each salmon fillet.

7. Bake in the oven for 16-22 minutes, or until the salmon is cooked through and the asparagus is tender.
8. Once cooked, remove from the oven and garnish with chopped parsley.

9. Serve hot and enjoy!

Nutritional Values per Person: Calories: 370 Total Fat: 23g Saturated Fat: 4g Cholesterol: 84 mg Sodium: 115mg Total Carbohydrate: 4g Dietary Fiber: 2g Sugar: 1g Protein: 36g

20. Lemon-Dill Grilled Salmon

Difficulty: Easy   **Preparation Time:** 12 minutes
Cooking Time: 10-12 minutes   **Serving:** 4

Ingredients:

- 4 salmon fillets (6 oz. each)
- 2 tbsps. olive oil
- Salt and pepper
- 1 lemon, sliced
- 2 tbsps. fresh dill, chopped
- 2 garlic cloves, minced

Instructions:

1. Heat the grill to medium-high heat.
2. Season the salmon with the oil, pepper and salt.
3. Skin side down, grill the salmon for 5-6 minutes.
4. Flip the salmon fillets and grill for an additional 5-6 minutes, or until the salmon is cooked through.
5. While the salmon is grilling, prepare the lemon and dill mixture by mixing together the chopped dill, minced garlic, and lemon slices in a small bowl.
6. Once the salmon is cooked, remove from the grill and place on a serving plate.
7. Spoon the lemon and dill mixture over the salmon fillets.
8. Serve hot and enjoy!

Nutritional Values per Person: Calories: 335 Total Fat: 20g Saturated Fat: 4g Cholesterol: 84 mg Sodium: 267 mg Total Carbohydrate: 3g Dietary Fiber: 1g Sugar: 1g Protein: 36g

121. Poached Salmon with Herbs

Difficulty: Easy   **Preparation Time:** 12 minutes

Cooking Time: 11-12 minutes   **Serving:** 4

Ingredients:

- 4 salmon fillets (6 oz. each)
- 4 cups of water
- 1/2 cup white wine
- 1 lemon, sliced
- 2 garlic cloves, minced
- 2 bay leaves
- 1 tbsp. fresh thyme leaves
- Salt and pepper

Instructions:

1. In a large pot, combine the water, white wine, lemon slices, garlic, bay leaves, thyme, salt, and pepper.
2. Bring everything to a boil.
3. Gently add the salmon fillets to the pot and reduce the heat to low.
4. Simmer the salmon fillets for 10-12 minutes, or until they are cooked through.
5. Once the salmon is cooked, remove the fillets from the pot using a slotted spoon and transfer to a serving dish.
6. Discard the lemon slices, bay leaves, and other solids from the poaching liquid.
7. Pour the poaching liquid over the salmon fillets.
8. Serve hot and enjoy!

Nutritional Values per Person: Calories: 259 Total Fat: 11g Saturated Fat: 2g Cholesterol: 83 mg Sodium: 134 mg Total Carbohydrate: 2g Dietary Fiber: 0g Sugar: 0g Protein: 34g

122. Baked Salt Cod Salad

Difficulty: Moderate   **Preparation Time:** 16 minutes (plus soaking time)

Cooking Time: 25-30 minutes   **Serving:** 4

Ingredients:

- 1 pound salt cod
- 1 red onion, thinly sliced
- 2 garlic cloves, minced
- 2 tbsps. olive oil
- 1/4 cup white wine vinegar
- 2 tbsps. chopped fresh parsley
- 2 tbsps. chopped fresh cilantro
- Salt and pepper, to taste
- 1 head Boston lettuce, washed and dried

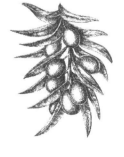

Instructions:

1. Soak the salt cod in cold water for at least 24 hours, changing the water several times.

2. Turn on the oven and bring it to 400°F (200°C).
3. In a baking dish, place the salt cod and cover with water.
4. Bake the salt cod for 25-32 minutes.
5. Remove the salt cod from the baking dish and let it cool slightly, then shred it into small pieces.
6. In a medium bowl, whisk together the red onion, garlic, oil, white wine vinegar, parsley, cilantro, pepper, and salt.
7. Add the shredded salt cod to the bowl and toss to combine.
8. Place a layer of Boston lettuce on a serving dish and spoon the salt cod salad on top.
9. Serve at room temperature and enjoy!

Nutritional Values per Person: Calories: 200 Total Fat: 7g Saturated Fat: 1g Cholesterol: 50 mg Sodium: 2200mg (Note: It's important to soak the salt cod to remove excess salt. Be sure to change the water several times.) Total Carbohydrate: 8g Dietary Fiber: 2g Sugar: 3g Protein: 25g

123. Salt Cod with Fennel and Tomatoes

Difficulty: Easy   **Preparation Time:** 16 minutes (plus soaking time)

Cooking Time: 30 minutes   **Serving:** 4

Ingredients:

- 1 pound salt cod
- 1 fennel bulb, sliced
- 1 pint cherry tomatoes
- 2 garlic cloves, minced
- 2 tbsps. olive oil, divided
- Salt and pepper, to taste

Instructions:

1. Soak the salt cod in cold water for at least 24 hours, changing the water several times.
2. Turn on the oven and bring it to 400°F (200°C).
3. In a large bowl, toss the fennel, cherry tomatoes, garlic, and 1 tbsp. of olive oil together.
4. Spread the vegetable mixture out in a baking dish.
5. Rinse the salt cod and pat it dry.
6. Place the salt cod on top of the vegetables and drizzle with the remaining olive oil.
7. Season everything with salt and pepper.
8. Bake for 25-30 minutes, or until the salt cod is cooked through and the vegetables are soft and beginning to caramelize.
10. Serve hot and enjoy!

Nutritional Values per Person: Calories: 200

Total Fat: 6g Saturated Fat: 1g Cholesterol: 50 mg Sodium: 1500mg (Note: It's important to soak the salt cod to remove excess salt. Be sure to change the water several times.) Total Carbohydrate: 12g Dietary Fiber: 4g Sugar: 6g Protein: 25g

124. Baked Salt Cod with Lemon and Oregano

Difficulty: Easy   **Preparation Time:** 16 minutes (plus soaking time)

Cooking Time: 30 minutes   **Serving:** 4

Ingredients:

- 1 pound salt cod
- 1 lemon, sliced
- 1/4 cup olive oil
- 2 cloves garlic, minced
- 1 tbsp. dried oregano
- Salt and pepper

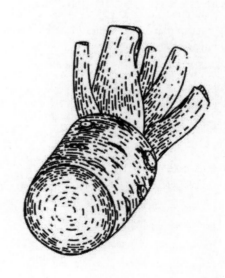

Instructions:

1. Soak the salt cod in cold water for at least 24 hours, changing the water several times.
2. Turn on the oven and bring it to 400°F (200°C).
3. In a bowl, whisk together the oil, minced garlic, and dried oregano.
4. Rinse the salt cod and pat it dry.
5. Place the salt cod in a baking dish and pour the olive oil mixture over the top.
6. Arrange the sliced lemon around the salt cod.
7. Season everything with pepper and salt.
8. Bake for 25-30 minutes, or until the salt cod is cooked through and the lemon slices are caramelized.
9. Serve hot and enjoy!

Nutritional Values per Person: Calories: 200 Total Fat: 6g Saturated Fat: 1g Cholesterol: 50 mg Sodium: 1500mg (Note: It's important to soak the salt cod to remove excess salt. Be sure to change the water several times.) Total Carbohydrate: 5g Dietary Fiber: 2g Sugar: 1g Protein: 30g

125. Salt Cod in Tomato Sauce

Difficulty: Medium   **Preparation Time:** 30 minutes (plus soaking time)

Cooking Time: 46 minutes   **Serving:** 4

Ingredients:

- 1 pound salt cod
- 1 can (14 ounces) crushed tomatoes
- 1 onion, chopped
- 2 cloves garlic, minced
- 2 tbsps. olive oil
- 1 tbsp. tomato paste
- 1 tsp dried oregano
- 1/4 tsp red pepper flakes
- Salt and pepper, to taste
- Fresh parsley, chopped

Instructions:

1. Soak the salt cod in cold water for at least 24 hours, changing the water several times.
2. In a Dutch oven or large saucepan, heat the oil over medium heat.
3. Add the chopped onion and cook about 5 minutes.
4. Add the minced garlic and cook for an additional minute.
5. Stir in the crushed tomatoes, tomato paste, dried oregano, and red pepper flakes.
6. Season with pepper and salt.
7. Simmer the sauce for 30 minutes, until it has slightly thickened.
8. Turn on the oven and bring it to 350°F (175°C).
9. Rinse the salt cod and pat it dry.
10. Cut the salt cod into bite-size pieces.
11. Add the salt cod to the tomato sauce and gently stir to coat.
12. Transfer the mixture to a baking dish and bake for 16-22 minutes.
13. Garnish with fresh parsley and serve hot.

Nutritional Values per Person: Calories: 200 Total Fat: 6g Saturated Fat: 1g Cholesterol: 50 mg Sodium: 1500mg (Note: It's important to soak the salt cod to remove excess salt. Be sure to change the water several times.) Total Carbohydrate: 12g Dietary Fiber: 3g Sugar: 7g Protein: 25g

126. Grilled Tuna Steaks with Lemon and Garlic

Difficulty: Easy   **Preparation Time:** 11 minutes

Cooking Time: 10 minutes   **Serving:** 4

Ingredients:

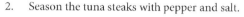

- 4 tuna steaks, about 6 ounces each
- 4 cloves garlic, minced
- 4 tbsps. olive oil
- 2 tbsps. lemon juice
- 1 tsp lemon zest
- Salt and pepper
- Lemon wedges, for serving

Instructions:

1. Turn the heat up and heat the grill over medium-high heat.
2. In a small bowl, combine the minced garlic, olive oil, lemon juice, and lemon zest.
3. Season the tuna steaks with pepper and salt on both sides.
4. Brush the garlic and lemon mixture onto both sides of each tuna steak.
5. Grill the tuna steaks for 3-5 minutes per side, or until they are heated through and have grill marks.
6. Serve the tuna steaks with lemon wedges on the side.

Nutritional Values per Person: Calories: 300 Total Fat: 16g Saturated Fat: 3g Cholesterol: 65 mg Sodium: 100mg Total Carbohydrate: 1g Dietary Fiber: 0g Sugar: 0g Protein: 36g

127. Seared Tuna Salad with Avocado

Difficulty: Intermediate   **Preparation Time:** 22 minutes

Cooking Time: 12 minutes   **Serving:** 2

Ingredients:

- 2 tuna steaks, about 6 ounces each
- 1 tbsp. olive oil
- Salt and pepper
- 4 cups mixed greens
- 1 avocado, sliced
- 1/2 cucumber, sliced
- 1/2 red onion, sliced
- 1/4 cup sliced almonds
- 2 tbsps. balsamic vinegar
- 1 tbsp. honey
- 1 tbsp. Dijon mustard

Instructions:

1. In a large skillet, heat the oil over medium-high heat.

2. Season the tuna steaks with pepper and salt.
3. Once the oil is hot, add the tuna steaks to the skillet and sear for 3-4 minutes per side, or until they are heated through and have a golden brown crust.
4. Remove the tuna and let it cool for 2-3 minutes.
5. In a bowl, toss together the mixed greens, sliced avocado, red onion and cucumber.
7. In a small bowl, whisk together the honey, balsamic vinegar, and Dijon mustard to make the dressing.
8. Divide the salad between two plates and top each with a tuna steak.
9. Drizzle the balsamic dressing over the salad and sprinkle the sliced almonds on top.

Nutritional Values per Person: Calories: 450 Total Fat: 27g Saturated Fat: 3.5g Cholesterol: 45mg Sodium: 220 mg Total Carbohydrate: 32g Dietary Fiber: 12g Sugar: 16g Protein: 30g

128. Grilled Tuna Kebabs with Vegetables

Difficulty: Intermediate   **Preparation Time:** 20 minutes

Cooking Time: 10-12 minutes   **Serving:** 4

Ingredients:

- 1 pound fresh tuna steak, cut into 1-inch cubes
- 2 tbsps. olive oil
- 2 tbsps. lemon juice
- Salt and pepper
- 1 red bell pepper, cut into 1-inch squares
- 1 green bell pepper, cut into 1-inch squares
- 1 red onion, cut into 1-inch squares
- 8 cherry tomatoes
- 8 skewers

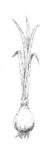

Instructions:

1. In a large bowl, whisk together the oil, salt, lemon juice, and pepper.
2. Add the cubed tuna to the bowl and toss to coat.
3. Let the tuna marinate for 12-16 minutes while you prepare the vegetables.
4. Preheat your grill to medium-high heat.
5. Thread the marinated tuna, bell peppers, onion, and cherry tomatoes onto the skewers, alternating the ingredients.
6. Grill the kebabs for 5-6 minutes per side, or until the tuna is cooked through and the vegetables are tender.
7. Remove the kebabs from the grill and let them rest for a few minutes before serving.

Nutritional Values per Person: Calories: 210 Total Fat: 10g Saturated Fat: 1.5g Cholesterol: 50 mg Sodium: 125 mg Total Carbohydrate: 7g Dietary Fiber: 1g Sugar: 4g Protein: 23g

129. Grilled Shrimp Tacos with Avocado Salsa

Difficulty: Intermediate   **Preparation Time:** 22 minutes

Cooking Time: 11-12 minutes   **Serving:** 4

Ingredients:

- 1 pound large shrimp, peeled and deveined
- 1 tbsp. olive oil
- 1 tsp chili powder
- 1/2 tsp garlic powder
- Salt and pepper
- 8 corn tortillas
- 1 ripe avocado, diced
- 1/2 red onion, diced
- 1 jalapeño pepper, seeded and finely chopped
- 1/4 cup chopped cilantro
- Juice of 1 lime
- Salt, to taste

Instructions:

1. Preheat your grill to medium-high heat.
2. In a bowl, combine the shrimp, oil, chili powder, garlic powder, salt, and pepper.
3. Thread the shrimp onto skewers and grill for 3-4 minutes per side.
4. Warm the corn tortillas on the grill for about 30 seconds per side.
5. In a medium bowl, mix together the diced avocado, red onion, jalapeño pepper, lime juice, cilantro and salt.
6. To assemble the tacos, add some grilled shrimp to each tortilla and top with a spoonful of avocado salsa.
7. Serve immediately and enjoy!

Nutritional Values per Person: Calories: 280 **Total Fat:** 10g **Saturated Fat:** 1.5g **Cholesterol:** 193mg **Sodium:** 320 mg **Total Carbohydrate:** 23g **Dietary Fiber:** 6g **Sugar:** 3g **Protein:** 27g

130. Steamed Cod with Vegetables in Lemon Broth

Difficulty: Easy   **Preparation Time:** 20 minutes

Cooking Time: 20 minutes   **Serving:** 4

Ingredients:

- 4 cod fillets
- 1 tbsp. olive oil
- 1 onion, chopped
- 2 garlic cloves, minced
- 2 cups chopped mixed vegetables (carrots, celery, zucchini or bell peppers)
- 4 cups low-sodium fish or vegetable broth
- 1 tbsp. lemon juice
- Salt and pepper

Instructions:

1. In a pot or skillet, heat oil over medium heat.
2. Add garlic and chopped onion and cook until softened, about 2-3 minutes.
3. Add mixed vegetables and cook for another 2-3 minutes until they begin to soften.
4. Add fish or vegetable broth and lemon juice to the pot, bring to a simmer.
5. Place cod fillets gently into the pot and lower the heat. Cover the pot and simmer for 8-10 minutes, or until the fish is cooked through and flakes easily with a fork.
6. Season with salt and pepper to taste.
7. Use a slotted spoon to remove the cod fillets from the pot and divide them among 4 plates.
8. Spoon the vegetables and lemon broth over the cod fillets and serve immediately.

Nutritional Values per serving: Calories: 180 **Total Fat:** 5g **Saturated Fat:** 1g **Cholesterol:** 50 mg **Sodium:** 330 mg **Total Carbohydrate:** 11g **Dietary Fiber:** 3g **Sugar:** 4g **Protein:** 24g

131. Grilled Halibut with Mango Salsa

Difficulty: Easy   **Preparation Time:** 10 minutes

Cooking Time: 15 minutes   **Serving:** 4

Ingredients:

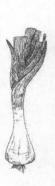

- 4 halibut fillets (about 6 ounces each)
- Salt and pepper
- 2 tbsps. olive oil
- 2 cups diced mango
- 1/2 cup diced red onion
- 1/4 cup chopped fresh cilantro
- 1 jalapeno, seeded and finely chopped
- Juice of 1 lime

Instructions:

1. Preheat grill to medium-high heat.
2. Season halibut fillets with pepper and salt to taste, and brush with oil.
3. Place the halibut on the grill and cook for 5-6 minutes on each side.
4. While the halibut is cooking, make the mango salsa. In a medium bowl, combine diced mango, red onion, cilantro, jalapeno, and lime juice. Mix well.
5. Once the halibut is done cooking, spoon the salsa over the fillets and serve hot.

Nutritional values per serving: Calories: 315 **Fat:** 12g **Carbs:** 20g **Fiber:** 3g **Protein:** 32g

132. Air Fry Crispy Shrimp Tacos

Difficulty: Intermediate   **Preparation Time:** 30 minutes
Cooking Time: 22 minutes   **Serving:** 4

Ingredients:

For the shrimp:

- 1 pound large shrimp, peeled and deveined
- 1/2 cup all-purpose flour
- 2 large eggs, beaten
- 1 cup panko breadcrumbs
- 1 tsp paprika
- 1/2 tsp garlic powder
- Salt and black pepper

For the tacos:

- 8 small corn tortillas
- 2 cups shredded cabbage
- 1 cup diced tomato
- 1/2 cup chopped fresh cilantro
- 1/4 cup diced red onion
- Juice of 1 lime
- Avocado, sliced (optional)

Instructions:

1. Preheat air fryer to 400°F.
2. Season the shrimp with black pepper and salt.
3. In three separate bowls, place the flour, eggs, and panko breadcrumbs mixed with paprika and garlic powder.
4. Dredge each shrimp in the flour, then dip into the egg mixture, and finally coat with the panko mixture. Repeat with remaining shrimp.
5. Arrange the shrimp in a single layer in the air fryer basket (you may have to work in batches). Spray lightly with cooking spray.
6. Air fry the shrimp for 10-12 minutes or until golden and crispy, flipping halfway through.
7. While the shrimp is cooking, mix the shredded cabbage, tomato, cilantro, red onion, and lime juice in a large bowl.
8. Warm the tortillas in a pan or in the microwave.
9. Assemble the tacos using the cooked shrimp and the cabbage mixture. Top with sliced avocado, if desired.

Nutritional values per serving:

- Calories: 320
- Fat: 10g
- Carbs: 32g
- Fiber: 5g
- Protein: 24g

133. Air Fry Lemon Pepper Cod

Difficulty: Easy   **Preparation Time:** 10 minutes
Cooking Time: 12 minutes   **Serving:** 2

Ingredients:

- 2 Cod fillets
- 1 lemon
- Salt and black pepper
- 1/2 tsp garlic powder
- 1/2 tsp paprika
- 1 tbsp. olive oil

Instructions:

1. Preheat air fryer to 400°F
2. Pat the cod fillets dry with paper towels.
3. Cut the lemon in half, and slice one half into thin rounds.
4. In a small bowl, mix together salt, black pepper, garlic powder, and paprika.
5. Brush the cod fillets with olive oil and sprinkle the spice mixture over both sides.
6. Place the cod fillets in the air fryer basket and arrange the lemon slices on top.
7. Air fry for 10-12 minutes or until the cod is cooked through and flakes easily with a fork.
8. Serve hot with additional lemon slices, if desired.

Nutritional values per serving: Calories: 220 **Fat:** 7g **Carbs:** 5g **Fiber:** 1g **Protein:** 34g

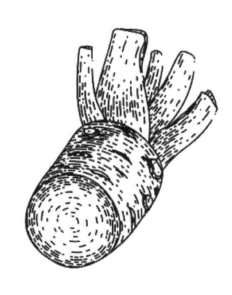

134. Garlic Butter Shrimp Linguine

Difficulty: Easy   **Preparation Time:** 12 minutes

Cooking Time: 22 minutes   **Serving:** 4

Ingredients:

- 8 oz. linguine
- 1 lb. raw shrimp, deveined and peeled
- 4 tbsps. unsalted butter
- 4 cloves garlic, minced
- 1/2 tsp red pepper flakes
- 1/4 cup chopped fresh parsley
- Black pepper and salt
- 1/4 cup grated Parmesan cheese

Instructions:

1. Cook the linguine according to package instructions until al dente.
2. While the pasta is cooking, heat butter in a large pan over medium heat.
3. Add garlic and red pepper flakes to the pan and cook, stirring frequently for 1-2 minutes or until fragrant.
4. Add the shrimp to pan and cook until pink and opaque, about 2-3 minutes per side.
5. Drain the pasta and mix it with the prawns in the pan.
6. Add chopped parsley and salt and pepper as needed.
7. Serve hot with a sprinkle of grated Parmesan cheese on top of each portion.

Nutritional values per serving: Calories: 393 Fat: 14g Carbs: 39g Fiber: 2g Protein: 27g

135. Lemon Herb Grilled Shrimp Skewers

Difficulty: Easy   **Preparation Time:** 16 minutes

Cooking Time: 8-10 minutes   **Serving:** 4

Ingredients:

- 1 lb. raw large shrimp, peeled and deveined
- 1/4 cup olive oil
- 2 tbsps. Chopped fresh parsley
- 2 tbsps. Chopped fresh basil
- 2 tbsps. chopped fresh thyme
- 2 cloves garlic, minced
- Juice of 1 lemon
- Salt and black pepper
- Wooden skewers, soaked in water for at least 30 minutes

Instructions:

1. Light the stove and heat the grill over medium-high heat

2. In a medium bowl, whisk together oil, minced garlic, chopped herbs, and lemon juice.
3. Add shrimp to the bowl, tossing to coat in the marinade.
4. Thread the shrimp onto wooden skewers.
5. Season the skewers with black pepper and salt.
6. Grill the skewers for 4 to 5 minutes per side, until the shrimp are pink.
7. Serve hot with additional lemon wedges and a sprinkle of chopped herbs on top.

Nutritional values per serving: Calories: 196 Fat: 12g Carbs: 2g Fiber: 0g Protein: 23g

136. Broiled Scallops with Lemon Butter Sauce

Difficulty: Easy   **Preparation Time:** 16 minutes

Cooking Time: 12 minutes   **Serving:** 4

Ingredients:

- 1 lb. scallops
- 1/4 cup unsalted butter, melted
- 2 cloves garlic, minced
- 2 tbsps. Lemon juice
- Black pepper and salt
- Lemon wedges, for serving

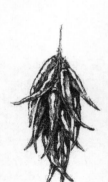

Instructions:

1. Preheat the broiler.
2. Rinse and pat dry the scallops.
3. In a bowl, whisk together melted butter, garlic, lemon juice, black pepper and salt.
4. Add scallops to the bowl and toss to coat in the butter mixture.
5. Arrange the scallops on a broiler pan.
6. Broil for 5-8 minutes, until the scallops are golden brown.
7. Serve hot with lemon wedges on the side.

Nutritional values per serving: Calories: 208 Fat: 14g Carbs: 1g Fiber: 0g Protein: 19g

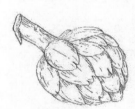

137. Seafood Stew with Tomatoes and Garlic

Difficulty: Medium   **Preparation Time:** 20 minutes

Cooking Time: 30 minutes   **Serving:** 6

Ingredients:

- 1 lb. assorted seafood (shrimp, scallops, mussels, and firm white fish), cleaned and deveined
- 1/4 cup olive oil
- 1 large onion, chopped
- 2 garlic cloves, minced
- 1 red bell pepper, seeded and chopped
- 1 can diced tomatoes
- 2 cups low-salt chicken broth
- 1/4 cup chopped fresh parsley
- Black pepper and salt

Instructions:

1. Heat the oil in a Dutch oven over medium heat.

2. Add garlic cloves and chopped onion and sauté for 5 minutes, until fragrant.

3. Add chopped red bell pepper and cook for an additional 6 minutes, until softened.

4. Add canned tomatoes and chicken broth to the pot.

5. Bring to a boil, then reduce the heat to low and simmer for 15 minutes.

6. Add assorted seafood to the pot and continue to cook for 5-7 minutes, until the seafood is cooked through.

7. Serve hot with a sprinkle of fresh parsley on top.

Nutritional values per serving: Calories: 254 Fat: 14g Carbs: 12g Fiber: 3g Protein: 22g

138. Poached Cod with Lemon Butter Sauce

Difficulty: Easy   **Preparation Time:** 12 minutes

Cooking Time: 15 minutes   **Serving:** 4

Ingredients:

- 4 cod fillets, about 6 oz. each
- 1/4 cup unsalted butter
- 2 cloves garlic, minced
- 2 tbsps. lemon juice
- 1/2 cup chicken broth
- Black pepper and salt
- Lemon wedges, for serving
- Fresh parsley, chopped for garnish

Instructions:

1. Melt the butter in a large skillet over medium heat.

2. Add garlic and cook for 1 minute, until fragrant.

3. Add lemon juice, chicken broth, black pepper and salt to the skillet and stir to combine.

4. Bring the mixture to a simmer.

5. Add the cod fillets to the skillet. Cover and poach the cod in the broth for 10-12 minutes, until cooked through.

6. Using a slotted spatula, carefully remove the cod from the skillet and place on a serving platter.

7. Spoon the lemon butter sauce over the cod fillets.

8. Garnish with chopped parsley and serve with lemon wedges on the side.

Nutritional values per serving: Calories: 230 Fat: 12g Carbs: 2g Fiber: 0g Protein: 28g

139. Grilled Swordfish Steaks with Mint Pesto

Difficulty: Intermediate   **Preparation Time:** 15 minutes

Cooking Time: 10-12 minutes   **Serving:** 4

Ingredients:

- 4 swordfish steaks, 6-8 oz. each
- 1/4 cup olive oil
- Black pepper and salt
- For the mint pesto:
- 1 cup fresh mint leaves
- 1/2 cup fresh parsley leaves
- 1/4 cup chopped walnuts
- 2 cloves garlic, minced
- 1/4 cup olive oil
- Black pepper and salt

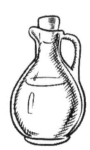

Instructions:

1. Light the burner and heat the grill over medium-high heat.

2. Rub the swordfish steaks with oil and season them with black pepper and salt.

3. Place the fish on the grill and cook it for 5-6 minutes on each side.

4. While the swordfish cooks, make the mint pesto. In a food processor, pulse the mint leaves, parsley leaves, chopped walnuts, minced garlic, olive oil, black pepper and salt until the mixture is smooth.

5. Serve the grilled swordfish steaks with a spoonful of mint pesto on top.

Nutritional values per serving: Calories: 415 Fat: 32g Carbs: 4g Fiber: 1g Protein: 29g

140. Pan-Seared Barramundi with Lemon and Capers

Difficulty: Easy **Preparation Time:** 12 minutes

Cooking Time: 11-12 minutes **Serving:** 4

Ingredients:

- 4 barramundi fillets, 6-8 oz. each
- 1/4 cup all-purpose flour
- Black pepper and salt
- 2 tbsp. olive oil
- 2 tbsp. unsalted butter
- 3 cloves garlic, minced
- 1/4 cup dry white wine
- 2 tbsp. fresh lemon juice
- 2 tbsp. capers
- 1 tbsp. chopped fresh parsley

Instructions:

1. Season the barramundi fillets with black pepper and salt, and coat them with flour, shaking off any excess.
2. In a skillet, heat olive oil and butter over medium heat. Once butter is melted, add the barramundi fillets and cook for 4-5 minutes.
4. Remove the barramundi fillets from the skillet and set aside.
5. Add minced garlic to the skillet and cook for 2 minutes until fragrant.
6. Pour in the white wine, lemon juice, and capers. Cook for 2-3 minutes until the wine reduces and the sauce thickens.
7. Return the barramundi fillets to the skillet and spoon the sauce over them. Cook for another minute until the fish is coated with sauce.
8. Serve the pan-seared barramundi fillets with chopped fresh parsley on top.

Nutritional values per serving: Calories: 294 Fat: 16g Carbs: 8g Fiber: 1g Protein: 24g

141. Grilled Mahi Mahi with Avocado and Tomato Salsa

Difficulty: Easy **Preparation Time:** 10 minutes

Cooking Time: 10 minutes **Serving:** 4

Ingredients:

- 4 mahi mahi fillets, 6-8 oz. each
- 1 tsp ground cumin
- 1 tsp smoked paprika
- Salt and black pepper
- 2 tbsp. olive oil
- 1 avocado, diced
- 1 large tomato, diced
- 1/4 red onion, finely chopped
- 1 jalapeño, seeded and minced
- 2 tbsp. chopped cilantro
- 2 tbsp. lime juice

Instructions:

1. Turn on the stove and heat a grill over medium-high heat
2. Season the mahi mahi fillets with ground cumin, smoked paprika, black pepper, and salt. Drizzle with oil.
9. Grill the mahi mahi fillets for 4-5 minutes on each side or until they are fully cooked and nicely charred.
10. In a separate bowl, mix together diced avocado, diced tomato, jalapeño, red onion, cilantro, and lime juice to make the avocado and tomato salsa.
11. Serve the grilled mahi mahi fillets with a generous scoop of avocado and tomato salsa on top.

Nutritional values per serving: Calories: 318 Fat: 21g Carbs: 13g Fiber: 7g Protein: 25g

142. Grilled Swordfish with Tomato Olive Relish

Difficulty: Easy **Preparation Time:** 12 minutes

Cooking Time: 12-15 minutes **Serving:** 4

Ingredients:

- 4 swordfish steaks, 6-8 oz. each
- Salt and black pepper
- 2 tbsp. olive oil
- 1 pint cherry tomatoes, halved
- 1/2 cup chopped kalamata olives
- 1/4 cup chopped fresh parsley
- 2 tbsp. red wine vinegar

Instructions:

1. Turn on the stove and heat a grill over medium-high heat.
2. Season the swordfish steaks with black pepper, salt, and oil.
3. Grill the swordfish steaks for 6-8 minutes on each side or until they are fully cooked and nicely charred.
4. In a separate bowl, mix together cherry tomatoes, kalamata olives, parsley, and red wine vinegar to make the tomato olive relish.
5. Top the grilled swordfish steaks with a generous scoop of tomato olive relish.

Nutritional values per serving: Calories: 306 Fat: 16g Carbs: 7g Fiber: 2g Protein: 35g

143. Seared Scallops with Spinach Salad

Difficulty: Moderate　　**Preparation Time:** 16 minutes

Cooking Time: 12 minutes　**Serving:** 4

Ingredients:

- 16 large sea scallops
- Salt and black pepper
- 2 tbsp. olive oil
- 6 cups fresh spinach leaves
- 1/4 cup chopped red onion
- 1/4 cup crumbled feta cheese
- 1/4 cup chopped fresh dill
- 2 tbsp. lemon juice
- 2 tbsp. honey

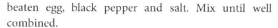

Instructions:

1. Season sea scallops with black pepper and salt.
2. Heat oil in a non-stick pan over high heat.
3. Add scallops to the hot pan and sear for 1-2 minutes on each side.
4. In a separate bowl, combine fresh spinach leaves, chopped red onion, crumbled feta cheese, and chopped fresh dill.
5. To make the dressing, mix lemon juice and honey in a small bowl.
6. Toss the spinach salad with the dressing until well coated.
7. Serve the seared scallops on top of the spinach salad.

Nutritional values per serving: Calories: 220 Fat: 10g Carbs: 10g Fiber: 2g Protein: 25g

144. Tuna Burger with Cucumber Yogurt Sauce

Difficulty: Easy　　**Preparation Time:** 16 minutes

Cooking Time: 12 minutes　**Serving:** 4

Ingredients:

- 2 cans of tuna, drained and flaked
- 1/2 cup breadcrumbs
- 1/4 cup chopped fresh parsley
- 1/4 cup chopped onion
- 1 egg, beaten
- Salt and black pepper
- 4 burger buns, toasted
- 1 small cucumber, grated
- 1/2 cup plain Greek yogurt
- 1 garlic clove, minced
- 1 tbsp. lemon juice
- Lettuce and tomato slices, for serving

Instructions:

1. In a mixing bowl, combine the drained and flaked tuna, breadcrumbs, chopped fresh parsley, chopped onion,

beaten egg, black pepper and salt. Mix until well combined.

2. Shape the tuna mixture into 4 patties.
3. Heat a non-stick pan or grill over medium heat. Add the tuna patties to the hot pan or grill and cook for 5-6 minutes on each side or until cooked through.
4. In a small mixing bowl, combine the grated cucumber, plain Greek yogurt, minced garlic, lemon juice, black pepper and salt. Mix until well combined.
5. Spread the cucumber yogurt sauce on the bottom half of each burger bun.
6. Top with a tuna patty, lettuce, tomato slices, and the top half of the burger bun.

Nutritional values per serving: Calories: 310 Fat: 6g Carbs: 30g Fiber: 2g Protein: 33g

145. Salmon Burger with Avocado Sauce

Difficulty: Easy　　**Preparation Time:** 10 minutes

Cooking Time: 12 minutes　**Serving:** 4

Ingredients:

- 1 lb. fresh salmon fillet, skin removed
- 2 tbsp. chopped red onion
- 2 garlic cloves, minced
- 1/4 cup chopped fresh cilantro
- 1 egg, beaten
- 1/2 cup breadcrumbs
- Salt and black pepper
- 4 burger buns, toasted
- 1 ripe avocado, pitted
- 1/4 cup plain Greek yogurt
- 1 tbsp. lime juice
- 1/2 tsp ground cumin
- Lettuce and tomato slices, for serving

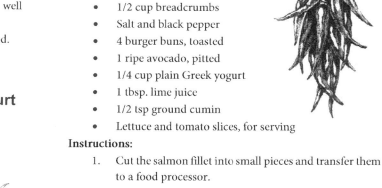

Instructions:

1. Cut the salmon fillet into small pieces and transfer them to a food processor.
2. Add chopped red onion, minced garlic, chopped fresh cilantro, beaten egg, breadcrumbs, black pepper and salt to the food processor. Pulse until well combined.
3. Shape the salmon mixture into 4 patties.
4. Heat a non-stick pan over medium heat. Add the salmon patties to the hot pan and cook for 4-5 minutes on each side.
5. In a separate bowl, mash the ripe avocado until smooth. Add plain Greek yogurt, lime juice, ground cumin, black pepper, and salt to the bowl. Mix until well combined.
6. Spread the avocado sauce on the bottom half of each burger bun.
7. Top with a salmon patty, lettuce, tomato slices, and the top half of the burger bun.

Nutritional values per serving: Calories: 390 Fat: 14g Carbs: 36g Fiber: 5g Protein: 29g

146. Grilled Mahi-Mahi Sandwich with Avocado and Tomato

Difficulty: Easy   **Preparation Time:** 15 minutes

Cooking Time: 10 minutes   **Serving:** 4

Ingredients:

- 1 lb. mahi-mahi fillet
- Salt and black pepper
- 1 tbsp. olive oil
- 4 burger buns, toasted
- 1 ripe avocado, sliced
- 1 large tomato, sliced
- 1/4 cup mayonnaise
- 1 tbsp. lemon juice
- 1 tbsp. chopped fresh cilantro
- Lettuce leaves, for serving

Instructions:

1. Turn up the heat and heat the grill over medium-high heat.
2. Season the mahi-mahi fillet with black pepper and salt. Drizzle with olive oil.
3. Grill the mahi-mahi fillet for 4-5 minutes on each side or until cooked through.
4. In a small mixing bowl, lemon juice, combine mayonnaise, chopped fresh cilantro, salt, and black pepper. Mix until well combined.
5. Spread the mayonnaise mixture on the bottom half of each burger bun.
6. Top with a grilled mahi-mahi fillet, sliced avocado, sliced tomato, lettuce leaves, and the top half of the burger bun.

Nutritional values per serving: Calories: 365 Fat: 17g Carbs: 28g Fiber: 7g Protein: 28g

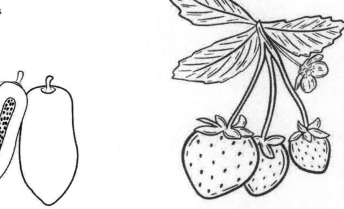

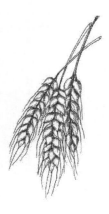

147. Tuna Salad Sandwich with Greek Yogurt and Celery

Difficulty: Easy   **Preparation Time:** 12 minutes

Cooking Time: N/A   **Serving:** 2

Ingredients:

- 1 can of tuna, drained
- 1/4 cup Greek yogurt
- 1/4 cup celery, finely chopped
- 1/4 cup red onion, finely chopped
- 1 tbsp. lemon juice
- 1 tbsp. chopped fresh parsley
- Salt and black pepper, to taste
- 4 slices of whole wheat bread
- Lettuce leaves, for serving

Instructions:

1. In a mixing bowl, combine drained tuna, Greek yogurt, chopped celery, chopped red onion, lemon juice, chopped fresh parsley, black pepper, and salt. Mix until well combined.
2. Toast the slices of whole wheat bread.
3. Spread the tuna salad mixture on two slices of toasted bread.
4. Add lettuce leaves on top of the tuna mixture.
5. Top with the other two slices of toasted bread.
6. Cut in half, serve, and enjoy your meal.

Nutritional values per serving: Calories: 250 Fat: 4g Carbs: 25g Fiber: 4g Protein:

148. Coconut Curry Fish Soup

Difficulty: Moderate   **Preparation Time:** 15 minutes

Cooking Time: 25 minutes   **Serving:** 4

Ingredients:

- 1 tbsp. olive oil
- 2 cloves of garlic, minced
- 1 tbsp. grated fresh ginger
- 2 tbsp. red curry paste
- 1 can of coconut milk
- 2 cups of fish stock
- 1 lb. firm white fish fillets, cut into small pieces
- 1 red bell pepper, chopped
- 1 zucchini, chopped
- 2 tbsp. chopped fresh cilantro
- Black pepper and salt

Instructions:

1. Heat the olive oil in a large pot over medium heat.
2. Add minced garlic, grated fresh ginger, and red curry paste. Cook for 1-2 minutes until fragrant.
3. Pour in the can of coconut milk and fish stock. Bring to a boil.
4. Add chopped red bell pepper and zucchini to the pot. Cook for 6-8 minutes until the vegetables are tender.
5. Add the small pieces of fish to the pot. Cook for 5-7 minutes until the fish is cooked through.
6. Season with black pepper and salt to taste.
7. Sprinkle chopped fresh cilantro over the top of the soup before serving.

Nutritional values per serving: Calories: 320 Fat: 23g

Carbs: 10g Fiber: 2g Protein: 21g

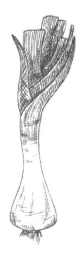

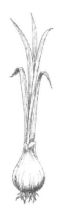

149. Steamed Fish with Ginger and Scallions

Difficulty: Easy   **Preparation Time:** 12 minutes

Cooking Time: 15 minutes   **Serving:** 4

Ingredients:

- 4 fillets of white fish (such as cod or haddock)
- 1-inch piece of ginger, peeled and sliced
- 3-4 scallions, sliced
- 2 tbsp. soy sauce (low-sodium)
- 1 tbsp. rice vinegar
- 1 tsp sesame oil
- Black pepper and salt
- Optional: steamed rice and stir-fried vegetables

Instructions:

1. Cut 4 pieces of parchment paper or aluminum foil into rectangles, large enough to wrap each fish fillet.
2. Season each fish fillet with salt and black pepper on both sides.
3. Place each seasoned fish fillet in the center of each parchment/foil rectangle.
4. Top each fillet with sliced ginger and scallions.
5. In a bowl, mix together rice vinegar, soy sauce, and sesame oil. Spoon the mixture over the top of each fish fillet.
6. Seal each parchment/foil rectangle tightly, folding the edges over several times to create a secure seal.
7. Place the wrapped fish in a steamer basket over boiling water. Cover and steam for 11-16 minutes until the fish is cooked through and opaque.
8. Carefully remove each fillet from the steamer basket and serve hot with steamed rice and stir-fried vegetables, if desired.

Nutritional values per serving: Calories: 150 Fat: 3g Carbs: 2g

Fiber: 1g Protein: 28g

150. Green Curry Fish

Difficulty: Intermediate   **Preparation Time:** 22 minutes

Cooking Time: 32 minutes   **Serving:** 4

Ingredients:

- 4 fillets of white fish (such as cod or tilapia)
- 1½ cups coconut milk (low-fat)
- 2 tbsp. green curry paste
- 1 tbsp. fish sauce
- 1 tbsp. brown sugar
- 1 red bell pepper, seeded and thinly sliced
- 1 small onion, thinly sliced
- 2 cloves garlic, minced
- 1 inch fresh ginger, grated
- 1 tbsp. vegetable oil
- 1 lime, cut into wedges
- Fresh cilantro leaves, for garnish
- Black pepper and salt

Instructions:

1. Season the fish with black pepper and salt.
2. In a large saucepan, heat the vegetable oil over medium-high heat.
3. Add the bell pepper and sliced onions to the skillet and sauté until soft, about 6 minutes.
4. Add the minced garlic and grated ginger to the skillet and sauté for another 1-2 minutes.
5. In a bowl, mix together the coconut milk, green curry paste, fish sauce, and brown sugar.
6. Add the coconut milk mixture to the skillet with the sautéed vegetables and bring to a simmer.
7. Add the seasoned fish fillets to the skillet, spooning the curry sauce over the fish.
8. Cover the skillet and let the fish cook in the sauce until opaque and cooked through, about 10-15 minutes.
9. Garnish with fresh cilantro leaves and serve hot with steamed rice and lime wedges on the side.

Nutritional values per serving: Calories: 300 Fat: 16g Carbs: 12g Fiber: 2g Protein: 24g

151. Tom Yum Soup with Fish

Difficulty: Easy   **Preparation Time:** 16 minutes

Cooking Time: 25 minutes   **Serving:** 4

Ingredients:

- 4 cups low-sodium chicken or fish broth
- 2 stalks lemongrass, outer layer removed and ends trimmed
- 3-4 kaffir lime leaves
- 3-4 Thai chilies, sliced (optional)
- 1-inch piece of galangal, sliced
- 1 small onion, sliced
- 2 cloves garlic, minced
- 1 tbsp. fish sauce
- 1 tbsp. brown sugar
- 2 cups mixed vegetables (such as sliced mushrooms, baby bok choy, snow peas, etc.)
- 4 fillets of white fish (such as cod or tilapia), cut into bite-sized pieces
- 2 tbsps. lime juice
- Fresh cilantro leaves, for garnish
- Black pepper and salt

Instructions:

1. In a large pot, bring the chicken or fish broth to a boil.
2. Reduce the heat to low and add the lemongrass, kaffir lime leaves, Thai chilies (if using), and sliced galangal. Let simmer for 12 minutes.
3. Add the onions and garlic to the pot and let simmer for another 5 minutes.
4. Add the fish sauce and brown sugar to the pot and stir well.
5. Add the mixed vegetables and let simmer for another 5-7 minutes, until the vegetables are tender.
6. Add the pieces of fish to the soup and simmer for 3-5 minutes, until the fish is cooked through.
7. Stir in the lime juice and season with salt and black pepper to taste.
8. Serve hot with fresh cilantro leaves as a garnish.

Nutritional values per serving: Calories: 180 Fat: 3g Carbs: 11g Fiber: 2g Protein: 28g

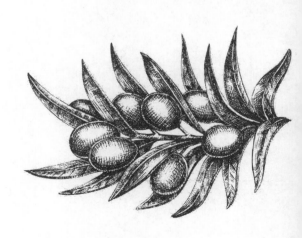

152. Hearty Fish Soup

Difficulty: Medium   **Preparation Time:** 30 minutes

Cooking Time: 1 hour 15 minutes   **Serving:** 6

Ingredients:

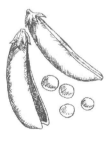

- 1 tbsp. olive oil
- 1 onion, chopped
- 2 cloves garlic, minced
- 1 fennel bulb, sliced
- 1 red pepper, chopped
- 1 yellow pepper, chopped
- 2 carrots, sliced
- 1 tsp smoked paprika
- 1 tsp ground cumin
- 1 tsp dried thyme
- 1 bay leaf
- Black pepper and salt
- 1 can (28 oz.) crushed tomatoes
- 4 cups low-sodium chicken or vegetable broth
- 2 cups water
- 6-8 small red potatoes, halved
- 1 pound white fish fillets, such as cod or haddock, cut into bite-sized pieces
- 2 tbsps. Fresh parsley, chopped
- Juice of 1 lemon

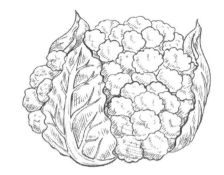

Instructions:

1. Heat the oil in a Dutch oven or saucepan
2. Add the garlic and onion and sauté until translucent.
3. Add the fennel, red and yellow peppers, and carrots to the pot and cook until they start to soften.
4. Add the smoked paprika, ground cumin, dried thyme, bay leaf, salt, and black pepper and stir well.
5. Pour in the crushed tomatoes, chicken or vegetable broth, and water. Stir to combine.
6. Add the potatoes and bring the soup to a boil.
7. Leave to boil for 45-50 minutes on a low flame.
8. Add the bite-sized fish pieces to the pot and cook for an additional 5-8 minutes or until the fish is cooked through.
9. Stir in the lemon juice and fresh parsley.
10. Serve hot with crusty bread or crackers.

Nutritional values per serving: Calories: 215 Fat: 4g Carbs: 30g Fiber: 8g Protein: 20

Salad

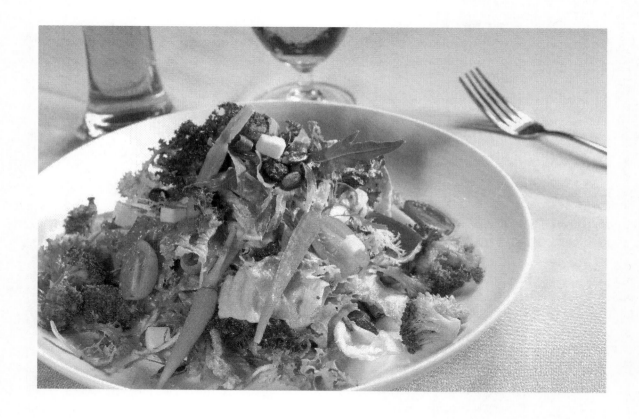

153. Greek Salad

Difficulty: Easy   **Preparation Time:** 15 minutes

Cooking Time: 0 minutes   **Serving:** 4

Ingredients:

- 1 head romaine lettuce, chopped
- 1/2 red onion, thinly sliced
- 1/2 English cucumber, diced
- 2 large tomatoes, diced
- 1 small green bell pepper, thinly sliced
- 1/2 cup pitted kalamata olives
- 1/2 cup crumbled feta cheese
- 2 tbsps. red wine vinegar
- 1/4 cup extra-virgin olive oil
- 1 tsp dried oregano
- Black pepper and salt

Instructions:

1. In a large serving bowl, add the chopped romaine lettuce.
2. Top the lettuce with the thinly sliced red onion, diced English cucumber, diced tomatoes, and thinly sliced green bell pepper.
3. Sprinkle the pitted kalamata olives and crumbled feta cheese over the top of the salad.
4. In a separate bowl, whisk together the red wine vinegar, extra-virgin olive oil, dried oregano, black pepper, and salt.
5. Drizzle the dressing over the salad and toss everything together until the salad is evenly coated with the dressing.
6. Serve immediately and enjoy!

Nutritional values per serving: Calories: 210 Fat: 17g Carbs: 10g Fiber: 3g Protein: 6g

154. Beet and Goat Cheese Salad

Difficulty: Easy   **Preparation Time:** 16 minutes

Cooking Time: 1 hour (to roast the beets)   **Serving:** 4

Ingredients:

- 4 medium beets, roasted and diced
- 4 cups mixed greens
- 4 oz. crumbled goat cheese
- 1/4 cup chopped walnuts
- 2 tbsp. extra-virgin olive oil
- 1 tbsp. red wine vinegar
- Pepper and salt

Instructions:

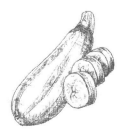

1. Preheat the oven to 400°F. Trim the ends off the beets and wrap them in foil.
2. Roast the beets in the oven for about 60 minutes.
3. Once the beets have cooled, peel and dice them into bite-sized pieces.
4. Divide the mixed greens onto four plates.
5. Top the mixed greens with the diced beets, crumbled goat cheese, and chopped walnuts.
6. In a bowl, whisk together the extra-virgin olive oil, red wine vinegar, pepper, and salt to create the dressing.
7. Drizzle the dressing over each serving of salad.
8. Enjoy!

Nutritional Values per Person: Calories: 250 Fat: 20g Carbohydrates: 10g Fiber: 3g Protein: 8g

155. Grilled Shrimp Salad

Difficulty: Medium   **Preparation Time:** 22 minutes

Cooking Time: 12 minutes   **Serving:** 4

Ingredients:

- 1 lb. large shrimp, peeled and deveined
- 1 tsp smoked paprika
- 1/2 tsp garlic powder
- Pepper and salt
- 4 cups mixed greens
- 1 avocado, diced
- 1/2 red onion, sliced
- 1/4 cup chopped cilantro
- 1/4 cup extra-virgin olive oil
- 2 tbsp. lime juice
- 1 tbsp. honey

Instructions:

1. In a bowl, combine the smoked paprika, salt, garlic powder, and pepper.
2. Season the shrimp with the spice mixture.
3. Place a grill pan or grill over medium-high heat
4. Grill the shrimp for 3-4 minutes per side.
5. In a bowl, combine the mixed greens, diced avocado, sliced red onion, and chopped cilantro.
6. In a bowl, whisk together the extra-virgin olive oil, lime juice, honey, pepper, and salt.
7. Pour and mix the dressing into the salad.
8. Divide the salad onto four plates and top with the grilled shrimp.
9. Enjoy!

Nutritional Values per Person: Calories: 300 Fat: 20g Carbohydrates: 15g Fiber: 6g Protein: 20g

156. Tuna Salad

Difficulty: Easy   **Preparation Time:** 12 minutes

Cooking Time: 0 minutes   **Serving:** 4

Ingredients:

- 2 cans of tuna in water, drained
- 4 cups mixed greens
- 4 small tomatoes, quartered
- 1/4 cup chopped red onion
- 1/4 cup chopped celery
- 2 tbsp. olive oil
- 1 tbsp. balsamic vinegar
- Pepper and salt

Instructions:

1. In a bowl, combine the drained tuna, mixed greens, quartered tomatoes, chopped red onion, and chopped celery.
2. In a bowl, whisk together the olive oil, salt, balsamic vinegar, and pepper to create the dressing.
3. Drizzle the dressing over the tuna salad and toss to coat.
4. Divide the tuna salad into four portions and serve.

Nutritional Values per Person: Calories: 220 Fat: 10g Carbohydrates: 9g Fiber: 2g Protein: 24g

157. Caprese Salad

Difficulty: Easy   **Preparation Time:** 12 minutes

Cooking Time: 0 minutes   **Serving:** 4

Ingredients:

- 2 large ripe tomatoes, sliced
- 8 oz. fresh mozzarella cheese, sliced
- 1/4 cup fresh basil leaves
- 2 tbsp. balsamic vinegar
- 1 tbsp. extra-virgin olive oil
- Salt and pepper, to taste

Instructions:

1. Arrange the sliced tomatoes and mozzarella on a platter, alternating them.
2. Add fresh basil leaves on top of the cheese and tomato slices.
3. In a bowl, whisk together the extra-virgin olive oil, balsamic vinegar, pepper, and salt.
5. Drizzle the dressing over the caprese salad.
6. Serve immediately.

Nutritional Values per Person: Calories: 180 Fat: 14g Carbohydrates: 4g Fiber: 1g Protein: 11g

158. Chicken Caesar Salad

Difficulty: Easy   **Preparation Time:** 15 minutes

Cooking Time: 15 minutes   **Serving:** 4

Ingredients:

- 2 chicken breasts, boneless and skinless
- Pepper and salt
- 1 tbsp. olive oil
- 8 cups chopped Romaine lettuce
- 1/2 cup grated Parmesan cheese
- 1/2 cup croutons
- Caesar dressing (homemade or store-bought)
- Lemon wedges (optional)

Instructions:

1. Turn on the oven and bring it to 375°F.
2. Season the chicken breasts with pepper and salt on both sides.
3. Place a frying pan over medium-high heat and heat the oil.
4. Add the chicken breasts and cook for about 7-8 minutes per side until browned and cooked through.
5. Remove the chicken from the pan and let it rest for 6 minutes before slicing.
6. In a large bowl, mix together the chopped Romaine lettuce, grated Parmesan cheese, and croutons.
7. Add the sliced chicken on top of the salad and drizzle with Caesar dressing.
8. Serve with lemon wedges on the side (optional).

Nutritional Values per Person: Calories: 320 Fat: 17g Carbohydrates: 10g Fiber: 3g Protein: 32g

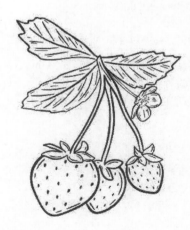

159. Waldorf Salad

Difficulty: Easy **Preparation Time:** 15 minutes

Cooking Time: 0 minutes **Serving:** 4

Ingredients:

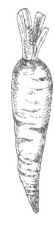

- 2 cups chopped apples
- 1 cup chopped celery
- 1/2 cup chopped walnuts
- 1/2 cup raisins
- 1/2 cup Greek yogurt
- 2 tbsp. honey
- 2 tbsp. lemon juice
- Pepper and salt
- 4 cups mixed salad greens

Instructions:

1. In a bowl, combine the chopped apples, celery, walnuts, and raisins.
2. In a separate bowl, mix together the Greek yogurt, lemon juice and honey, until well combined.
3. Pour the yogurt dressing over the apple mixture and stir well to combine.
4. Season with salt and pepper.
5. Divide the mixed salad greens onto 4 plates or bowls.
6. Top each bed of greens with an equal amount of the apple mixture.
7. Serve immediately.

Nutritional Values per Person: Calories: 250 Fat: 11g Carbohydrates: 39g Fiber: 5g Protein: 7g

160. Egg Salad

Difficulty: Easy **Preparation Time:** 12 minutes

Cooking Time: 12 minutes **Serving:** 4

Ingredients:

- 6 hard-boiled eggs, peeled and chopped
- 1/4 cup diced red onion
- 1/4 cup diced celery
- 2 tbsp. plain Greek yogurt
- 1 tbsp. mayonnaise
- 1 tbsp. Dijon mustard
- 1 tbsp. chopped fresh dill
- Black pepper and salt
- 4 cups mixed salad greens

Instructions:

1. In a medium bowl, combine the chopped hard-boiled eggs, red onion, and celery.

2. In another bowl, whisk together the Greek yogurt, mayonnaise, Dijon mustard, and chopped dill until well blended.
3. Pour the dressing over the egg mixture and mix well to combine.
4. Season with black pepper and salt.
5. To assemble the salad, divide the mixed salad greens equally onto 4 plates or bowls.
6. Top each bed of greens with an equal amount of the egg salad mixture.
7. Serve immediately.

Nutritional Values per Person: Calories: 200 Fat: 13g Carbohydrates: 4g Fiber: 2g Protein: 15g

161. Spinach Salad

Difficulty: Easy **Preparation Time:** 17 minutes

Cooking Time: None **Serving:** 4

Ingredients:

- 6 cups baby spinach leaves
- 1/2 cup sliced red onion
- 1/2 cup sliced mushrooms
- 1/2 cup cherry tomatoes, halved
- 1/4 cup crumbled feta cheese
- 1/4 cup sliced almonds
- 2 tbsp. balsamic vinegar
- 2 tbsp. extra-virgin olive oil
- 1 tsp Dijon mustard
- Black pepper and salt

Instructions:

1. In a large salad bowl, toss together the baby spinach, red onion, mushrooms, cherry tomatoes, feta cheese, and sliced almonds.

2. In a small bowl, whisk together the extra-virgin olive oil, balsamic vinegar, Dijon mustard, black pepper and salt until well blended.

3. Drizzle the dressing over the salad and toss well to coat all the ingredients.

4. Serve immediately.

Nutritional Values per Person: Calories: 150 Fat: 11g Carbohydrates: 8g Fiber: 3g Protein: 5g

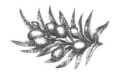

162. Quinoa Salad

Difficulty: Easy   **Preparation Time:** 22 minutes

Cooking Time: 17 minutes   **Serving:** 4

Ingredients:

- 1 cup quinoa
- 2 cups water
- 1 red bell pepper, diced
- 1 yellow bell pepper, diced
- 1 cucumber, diced
- 1/2 red onion, diced
- 1/2 cup fresh parsley, chopped
- 1/4 cup fresh mint, chopped
- 1/4 cup extra-virgin olive oil
- 2 tbsp. red wine vinegar
- 1 tsp. Dijon mustard
- Salt and black pepper, to taste

Instructions:

1. In a medium saucepan, bring the quinoa and water to a boil. Reduce heat to low and simmer for 17 minutes.
2. Remove from heat and transfer the quinoa to a large salad bowl. Let it cool.
3. Add the diced bell peppers, red onion, cucumber, parsley, and mint to the quinoa.
4. In a bowl, whisk together the olive oil, red wine vinegar, Dijon mustard, salt, and black pepper until well blended.
5. Drizzle the dressing over the salad and toss well to coat all the ingredients.
6. Serve chilled.

Nutritional Values per Person: Calories: 270 Fat: 14g Carbohydrates: 31g Fiber: 5g Protein: 6g

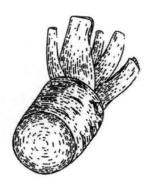

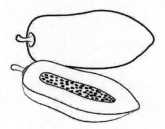

163. Fatty Liver Fighting Salad

Difficulty: Easy   **Preparation Time:** 20 minutes

Cooking Time: 0 minutes   **Serving:** 2 persons

Ingredients:

- 2 cups mixed greens (spinach, arugula, and romaine lettuce)
- 1 cup diced watermelon
- 1 cup diced mango
- 1/4 cup slivered almonds
- 1/4 cup crumbled goat cheese
- 2 tbsp. balsamic vinegar
- 1 tbsp. extra-virgin olive oil
- Pepper and salt

Instructions:

1. Begin by rinsing the mixed greens thoroughly and patting them dry with paper towels.
2. In a bowl, toss the mixed greens, diced watermelon, and diced mango together until combined.
3. In a mixing bowl, whisk together the extra-virgin olive oil, balsamic vinegar, pepper. and salt to create the balsamic vinaigrette.
4. Drizzle the vinaigrette over the salad and gently toss everything together to combine.
5. Sprinkle the slivered almonds and crumbled goat cheese over the top of the salad, and give everything one final gentle toss.
6. Divide the salad evenly between two plates and serve immediately.

Nutritional Values Per Person: Calories 234 Fat 15.2g Carbohydrates 18.5g Fiber 3.3g Protein 7.5g

Dessert

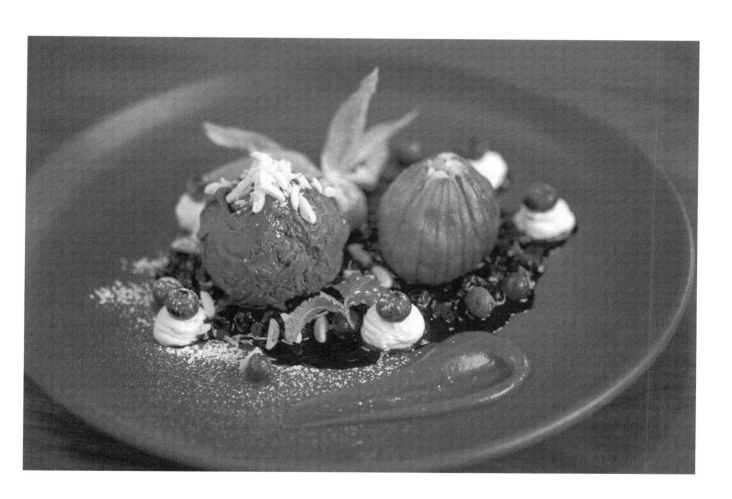

164. Baked Apples

Difficulty: Easy   **Preparation Time:** 12 minutes
Cooking Time: 45 minutes   **Serving:** 4

Ingredients:

- 4 large apples
- 2 tbsp. of honey
- 2 tbsp. of coconut oil
- 1/2 tsp of ground cinnamon
- 1/4 cup of chopped almonds
- 1/4 cup of raisins

Instructions:

1. Turn on the oven and bring it to 375°F.
2. Cut a thin slice off the top of each apple, then use a spoon or melon baller to scoop out the core, leaving about 1/2 inch at the bottom.
3. In a bowl, mix together honey, melted coconut oil, and ground cinnamon.
4. Fill each apple with the honey mixture and place them in a baking dish.
5. Sprinkle the chopped almonds and raisins over the top of each apple.
6. Bake until the apples are tender and the filling is caramelized, about 40 to 45 minutes.
7. Remove from the oven and let them cool for 6 minutes before serving.

Nutritional Values per Person: Calories: 200 Fat: 8g Carbohydrates: 34g Fiber: 6g Protein: 2g

165. Fruit Salad

Difficulty: Easy   **Preparation Time:** 15 minutes
Cooking Time: 0 minutes   **Serving:** 4

Ingredients:

- 2 cups diced fresh pineapple
- 2 cups diced fresh strawberries
- 2 cups diced fresh mango
- 1/2 cup blueberries
- 1/4 cup chopped fresh mint leaves
- 2 tbsp. honey
- 2 tbsp. freshly squeezed lime juice
- Optional: 1/4 cup chopped walnuts or almonds

Instructions:

1. In a bowl, combine the diced pineapple, strawberries, mango, and blueberries.
2. Add in the chopped fresh mint leaves and mix well.
3. In a bowl, whisk the lime juice and honey until well blended.

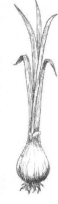

4. Drizzle the dressing over the fruit mixture and toss well to coat all the ingredients.
5. Optional: sprinkle the chopped walnuts or almonds over the fruit salad just before serving.

Nutritional Values per Person: Calories: 175 Fat: 2g Carbohydrates: 43g Fiber: 6g Protein: 3g

166. Chocolate Banana Smoothie

Difficulty: Easy   **Preparation Time:** 6 minutes
Cooking Time: 0 minutes   **Serving:** 2

Ingredients:

- 2 ripe bananas, peeled and sliced
- 1 cup almond milk
- 2 tbsp. unsweetened cocoa powder
- 1 tbsp. honey
- 1 tsp vanilla extract
- 1 cup ice cubes

Instructions:

1. In a blender, combine the sliced bananas, cocoa powder, almond milk, honey, and vanilla extract.
2. Add in the ice cubes and blend until smooth and creamy.
3. Pour the smoothie into two glasses and serve immediately.

Nutritional Values per Person: Calories: 125 Fat: 3g Carbohydrates: 27g Fiber: 4g Protein: 2g

167. Tutti-Frutti Smoothie

Difficulty: Easy   **Preparation Time:** 6 minutes
Cooking Time: 0 minutes   **Serving:** 2

Ingredients:

- 1 cup mixed berries (fresh or frozen)
- 1 banana, peeled and sliced
- 1 cup almond milk
- 1 tbsp. honey
- 1 tsp vanilla extract
- 1 cup ice cubes

Instructions:

1. Combine the mixed berries, sliced banana, almond milk, honey, and vanilla extract in a blender.
2. Add in the ice cubes and blend until smooth and creamy.
3. Pour the smoothie into two glasses and serve immediately.

Nutritional Values per Person: Calories: 120 Fat: 2g Carbohydrates: 26g Fiber: 5g - Protein: 2g

168. Berry Sorbet

Difficulty: Moderate   **Preparation Time:** 10 minutes

Cooking Time: 0 minutes   **Serving:** 4

Ingredients:

- 2 cups mixed berries (fresh or frozen)
- 1/2 cup water
- 1/2 cup sugar
- 1 tbsp. lemon juice

Instructions:

1. Heat the sugar and water in a small saucepan, stir until the sugar is completely dissolved.
2. Add the mixed berries and lemon juice to a blender and blend until smooth.
3. Pour the berry mixture into the saucepan with the sugar syrup and mix well.
4. Let the mixture cool in the refrigerator for at least 1 hour.
5. Pour the berry mixture into an ice cream maker and shake according to the manufacturer's instructions.
6. Once the sorbet is done, transfer it to a freezer-safe container and freeze for at least 1 hour before serving.

Nutritional Values per Person: Calories: 100 Fat: 0g Carbohydrates: 26g Fiber: 2g Protein: 0g

169. Apple Crisp

Difficulty: Easy   **Preparation Time:** 20 minutes

Cooking Time: 35-40 minutes   **Serving:** 6

Ingredients:

- 6 cups sliced apples
- 1/2 cup all-purpose flour
- 1/2 cup rolled oats
- 1/2 cup brown sugar
- 1/2 cup unsalted butter, softened
- 1 tsp cinnamon
- 1/4 tsp nutmeg

Instructions:

1. Turn on the oven and bring it to 350°F (175°C). Grease a 9x13 inch baking pan.
2. Arrange the sliced apples in the prepared pan.
3. In a separate bowl, mix together the flour, rolled oats, brown sugar, butter, cinnamon, and nutmeg until crumbly.
4. Sprinkle the crumb mixture over the apples.
5. Bake for 36-42 minutes or until the topping is golden brown and the apples are tender.
6. Serve warm with vanilla ice cream or whipped cream, if desired.

Nutritional Values per Person: Calories: 332 Fat: 16g Carbohydrates: 47g Fiber: 5gYProtein: 2g

170. Banana Oat Cookies

Difficulty: Easy   **Preparation Time:** 12 minutes

Cooking Time: 16-22 minutes   **Serving:** 12

Ingredients:

- 2 ripe bananas, mashed
- 1 1/2 cups rolled oats
- 1/4 cup almond butter1/4 cup honey
- 1/2 tsp cinnamon
- Pinch of salt

Instructions:

1. Turn on the oven and bring it to 350°F (175°C). Line a baking sheet with parchment paper.
2. In a bowl, mix together the mashed bananas, rolled oats, almond butter, honey, cinnamon, and salt until well combined.
3. Drop spoonfuls of the mixture onto the prepared baking sheet.
4. Bake for 15-20 minutes, or until the cookies are golden brown.
5. Transfer to a wire rack to cool completely.

Nutritional Values per Person: Calories: 110 Fat: 3g Carbohydrates: 19g Fiber: 2g Protein: 3g

171. Green Yogurt and Mixed Berries Bowl

Difficulty: Easy   **Preparation Time:** 12 minutes

Cooking Time: N/A   **Serving:** 1

Ingredients:

- 1/2 cup plain Greek yogurt
- 1/2 ripe avocado
- 1 tbsp. honey
- 1/2 tsp vanilla extract
- 1/2 cup mixed berries (such as blueberries, strawberries, and raspberries)
- 1 tbsp. chopped almonds or pistachios
- Fresh mint leaves for garnish

Instructions:

1. In a blender, blend together the Greek yogurt, avocado, honey, and vanilla extract until smooth.
2. Transfer the mixture to a bowl.
3. Top with the mixed berries and chopped nuts.
4. Garnish with fresh mint leaves.

Nutritional Values per Person: Calories: 362 Fat: 18g Carbohydrates: 36g Fiber: 10g Protein: 20g

172. Chocolate Chia Pudding

Difficulty: Easy   **Preparation Time:** 12 minutes
Cooking Time: N/A   **Serving:** 2

Ingredients:

- 1/4 cup chia seeds
- 1 cup unsweetened almond milk
- 2 tbsp. unsweetened cocoa powder
- 1-2 tbsp. honey or maple syrup
- 1/2 tsp vanilla extract
- Pinch of sea salt
- Fresh berries for garnish

Instructions:

1. In a medium-sized bowl, whisk together chia seeds, almond milk, cocoa powder, honey or maple syrup, vanilla extract, and sea salt.
2. Whisk until everything is well combined and there are no lumps.
3. Cover the bowl and refrigerate for at least 2 hours, or until the mixture thickens.
4. Stir occasionally to prevent clumps from forming.
5. Once thickened, divide the pudding into two separate cups or bowls.
6. Garnish with fresh berries before serving.

Nutritional Values per Person: Calories: 180 Fat: 8g Carbohydrates: 25g Fiber: 11g Protein: 6g

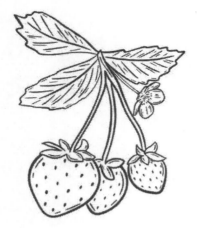

173. Blueberry and Almond Flour Muffins

Difficulty: Easy   **Preparation Time:** 15 minutes
Cooking Time: 26 minutes   **Serving:** 8 muffins

Ingredients:

- 2 cups almond flour
- 1/4 cup honey
- 1 tsp baking powder
- 1/2 tsp baking soda
- 1/2 tsp sea salt
- 2 large eggs
- 1/4 cup unsweetened almond milk
- 1/4 cup coconut oil, melted
- 1 tsp vanilla extract
- 1 cup fresh blueberries

Instructions:

1. Turn on the oven and bring it to 350°F/ 180°C and line a muffin tin with eight muffin liners.
2. In a mixing bowl, whisk together almond flour, baking powder, baking soda, and sea salt.
3. Add honey, eggs, almond milk, melted coconut oil, and vanilla extract to the bowl and stir until everything is well combined.
4. Add fresh blueberries to the mixture and gently stir until evenly distributed.
5. Spoon batter into the muffin liners, filling them about three-quarters full.
6. Bake for 25 minutes, or until a toothpick inserted in the middle of a muffin comes out clean.
7. Let the muffins cool in the tin for a few minutes before transferring them to a cooling rack.

Nutritional Values per Person: Calories: 250 Fat: 21g Carbohydrates: 12g Fiber: 3g Protein: 7g

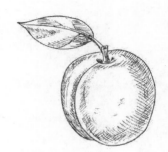

Vegetable and Fruit Juices

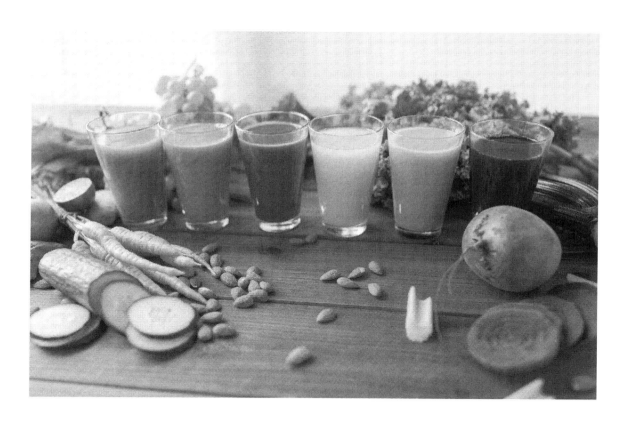

174. Green Detox Juice

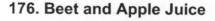

Difficulty: Easy   **Preparation Time:** 10 minutes

Cooking Time: 0 minutes   **Serving:** 1 serving

Ingredients:

- 1/2 cucumber
- 1 green apple
- 1 small handful of spinach
- 1 small handful of kale1/2 lemon, peeled
- 1 inch of fresh ginger root
- 1 cup of water

Instructions:

1. Wash all of the fruits and vegetables and cut them into small chunks.
2. Add the cucumber, apple, spinach, kale, lemon, and ginger to a blender.
3. Add one cup of water to the blender and blend on high until the juice is smooth.
4. Pour the juice into a glass and enjoy immediately.

Nutritional Values per Person: Calories: 110 Fat: 0.5g Carbohydrates: 28g Fiber: 8g Protein: 3g

175. Carrot and Ginger Juice

Difficulty: Easy   **Preparation Time:** 10 minutes

Cooking Time: 0 minutes   **Serving:** 2 servings

Ingredients:

- 4 large carrots
- 1 inch of fresh ginger root1/2 lemon, peeled
- 1 cup of water

Instructions:

1. Wash the carrots and ginger root and cut them into small chunks.
2. Add the carrots, ginger, and lemon to a blender.
3. Add one cup of water to the blender and blend on high until the juice is smooth.
4. Pour the juice into glasses and serve immediately.

Nutritional Values per Person: Calories: 60 Fat: 0.5g Carbohydrates: 14g Fiber: 4g Protein: 2g

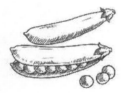

176. Beet and Apple Juice

Difficulty: Easy   **Preparation Time:** 10 minutes

Cooking Time: 0 minutes   **Serving:** 2 servings

Ingredients:

- 2 small beets
- 1 large apple
- 1 inch of fresh ginger root
- 1/2 lemon, peeled
- 1 cup of water

Instructions:

1. Wash the beets, apple, and ginger root.
2. Cut the beets and apple into small chunks.
3. Add the beets, apple, ginger, and lemon to a blender.
4. Add one cup of water to the blender and blend on high until the juice is smooth.
5. Pour the juice into glasses and serve immediately.

Nutritional Values per Person: Calories: 100 Fat: 0.5g Carbohydrates: 25g Fiber: 5g Protein: 2g

177. Pineapple and Kale Juice

Difficulty: Easy   **Preparation Time:** 12 minutes

Cooking Time: 0 minutes   **Serving:** 2 servings

Ingredients:

- 1 cup fresh pineapple
- 2 cups kale
- 1/2 cucumber
- 1/2 lemon, peeled
- 1 tsp honey
- 1 cup of water

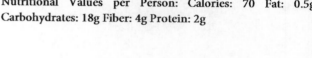

Instructions:

1. Wash the kale, cucumber, and pineapple.
2. Cut the pineapple into small chunks.
3. Add the kale, cucumber, pineapple, lemon, honey, and one cup of water to a blender.
4. Blend the ingredients on high until the juice is smooth.
5. Pour the juice into glasses and serve.

Nutritional Values per Person: Calories: 70 Fat: 0.5g Carbohydrates: 18g Fiber: 4g Protein: 2g

178. Turmeric and Orange Juice

Difficulty: Easy   **Preparation Time:** 12 minutes

Cooking Time: 0 minutes   **Serving:** 2 servings

Ingredients:

- 2 oranges, peeled
- 1 small piece of fresh turmeric, peeled
- 1 small piece of fresh ginger, peeled
- 1/4 tsp black pepper
- 1 tsp honey
- 1 cup of water

Instructions:

1. Cut the oranges into small chunks.
2. Add the oranges, turmeric, ginger, black pepper, honey, and one cup of water to a blender.
3. Blend the ingredients on high until the juice is smooth.
4. Pour the juice into glasses and serve.

Nutritional Values per Person: Calories: 70 Fat: 0.5g Carbohydrates: 18g Fiber: 4g Protein: 2g

179. Watermelon and Mint Juice

Difficulty: Easy   **Preparation Time:** 12 minutes

Cooking Time: 0 minutes   **Serving:** 4 servings

Ingredients:

- 4 cups fresh watermelon cubes, seeds removed
- 10 fresh mint leaves, washed
- Juice of 1 lime
- 1 tbsp. honey
- 1 cup of water
- Ice cubes (optional)

Instructions:

1. Add the watermelon cubes, mint leaves, lime juice, honey, and one cup of water to a blender.
2. Blend the ingredients on high until the juice is smooth.
3. If desired, add ice cubes to the blender and blend for a few seconds to make the juice cold and frothy.
4. Pour the juice into glasses and serve.

Nutritional Values per Person: Calories: 60 Fat: 0.5g Carbohydrates: 15g Fiber: 1g Protein: 1g

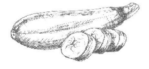

180. Green Apple and Cucumber Juice

Difficulty: Easy   **Preparation Time:** 12 minutes

Cooking Time: 0 minutes   **Serving:** 2 servings

Ingredients:

- 1 green apple, cored and sliced
- 1/2 cucumber, sliced
- 2 stalks celery, sliced
- 1 handful fresh spinach
- 1 small piece of ginger, peeled and grated
- 1/2 lemon, juiced
- 1 cup of water
- Ice cubes (optional)

Instructions:

1. Add the apple, cucumber, celery, spinach, ginger, lemon juice, and one cup of water to a blender.
2. Blend the ingredients on high until the juice is smooth.
3. If desired, add ice cubes to the blender and blend for a few seconds to make the juice cold and frothy.
4. Pour the juice into glasses and serve.

Nutritional Values per Person: Calories: 80 Fat: 0.5g Carbohydrates: 19g Fiber: 4g Protein: 2g

181. Citrus Burst Juice

Difficulty: Easy   **Preparation Time:** 12 minutes

Cooking Time: 0 minutes   **Serving:** 2 servings

Ingredients:

- 2 medium oranges, peeled and segmented
- 1 grapefruit, peeled and segmented
- 1 lemon, juiced
- 1 tbsp. honey
- 1 inch fresh ginger root, peeled
- Ice cubes (optional)

Instructions:

1. Add the oranges, grapefruit, lemon juice, honey, and ginger root to a juicer or blender.
2. Blend the ingredients on high until the juice is smooth.
3. If desired, add ice cubes to the blender and blend for a few seconds to make the juice cold and frothy.
4. Pour the juice into glasses and serve.

Nutritional Values per Person: Calories: 110 Fat: 0.5g Carbohydrates: 28g Fiber: 4g Protein: 2g

182. Carrot and Pineapple Juice

Difficulty: Easy **Preparation Time:** 10 minutes
Cooking Time: 0 minutes **Serving:** 2 servings
Ingredients:

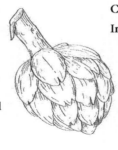

- 2 large carrots, peeled and chopped
- 2 cups of fresh pineapple, chopped
- 1 tbsp. of honey
- 1/2 inch piece of ginger, peeled and grated
- 1/2 cup of water
- Ice cubes (optional)

Instructions:

1. Add the chopped carrots, pineapple, honey, ginger, and water to a blender.
2. Blend the ingredients at a high speed until the juice is smooth.
3. If desired, add ice cubes to the blender and blend for a few seconds to make the juice cold and frothy.
4. Pour the juice into glasses and serve.

Nutritional Values per Person: Calories: 100 Fat: 0.5g Carbohydrates: 25g Fiber: 4g Protein: 2g

183. Berry Blast Juice

Difficulty: Easy **Preparation Time:** 10 minutes
Cooking Time: 0 minutes **Serving:** 2 servings
Ingredients:

- 1 cup of mixed berries (strawberries, blueberries, raspberries)
- 1 banana, peeled and chopped
- 1/2 cup of low-fat yogurt
- 1/2 cup of unsweetened almond milk
- 1 tsp of honey
- Ice cubes (optional)

Instructions:

1. Add the mixed berries, chopped banana, low-fat yogurt, almond milk, and honey to a blender.
2. Blend the ingredients at a high speed until the juice is smooth.
3. If desired, add ice cubes to the blender and blend for a few seconds to make the juice cold and frothy.
4. Pour the juice into glasses and serve.

Nutritional Values per Person: Calories: 150 Fat: 3g Carbohydrates: 30g Fiber: 6g Protein: 6g

184. Citrus Ginger Morning Juice

Difficulty: Easy **Preparation Time:** 12 minutes
Cooking Time: 0 minutes **Serving:** 2 servings
Ingredients:

- 2 oranges, peeled and divided into segments
- 1 grapefruit, peeled and divided into segments
- 1 inch of fresh ginger, peeled and chopped
- 1/4 cup of fresh mint leaves
- 1/4 cup of water
- Ice cubes (optional)

Instructions:

1. Add the oranges, grapefruit, ginger, and mint leaves to a blender.
2. Blend the ingredients at a high speed until they are well mixed.
3. Add 1/4 cup of water to the blender and blend for a few more seconds until you get the desired consistency.
4. If desired, add ice cubes to the blender and blend for a few seconds to make the juice cold and frothy.
5. Pour the juice into glasses and serve.

Nutritional Values per Person: Calories: 70 Fat: 0.5g Carbohydrates: 17g Fiber: 4g Protein: 1.5g

185. Beet and Carrot Juice

Difficulty: Easy **Preparation Time:** 16 minutes
Cooking Time: 0 minutes **Serving:** 2 servings
Ingredients:

- 1 medium beet, peeled and chopped
- 2 medium carrots, peeled and chopped
- 1/2 inch of fresh ginger, peeled and chopped
- 1/2 lemon, juiced
- 1 cup of water
- Ice cubes (optional)

Instructions:

1. Add the chopped beet, carrots, and ginger to a blender.
2. Blend the ingredients at a high speed until they are well mixed.
3. Add 1 cup of water to the blender and blend for a few more seconds until you get the desired consistency.
4. Add fresh lemon juice to the blender and blend for a few more seconds.
5. If desired, add ice cubes to the blender and blend for a few seconds to make the juice cold and frothy.
6. Pour the juice into glasses and serve.

Nutritional Values per Person: Calories: 70 Fat: 0.5g Carbohydrates: 17g Fiber: 4g Protein: 1.5g

186. Tangy Green Juice

Difficulty: Easy **Preparation Time:** 10 minutes

Cooking Time: 0 minutes **Serving:** 2 servings

Ingredients:

- 1 cucumber, chopped
- 1 green apple, chopped
- 1 handful of fresh baby spinach
- 1/2 lemon, juiced
- 1/2 inch of fresh ginger, peeled and chopped
- 1 cup of water
- Ice cubes (optional)

Instructions:

1. Add the chopped cucumber, green apple, and baby spinach to a blender.
2. Blend the ingredients at a high speed until they are well mixed.
3. Add 1 cup of water to the blender and blend for a few more seconds until you get the desired consistency.
4. Add fresh lemon juice and chopped ginger to the blender and blend for a few more seconds.
5. If desired, add ice cubes to the blender and blend for a few seconds to make the juice cold and frothy.
6. Pour the juice into glasses and serve.

Nutritional Values per Person: **Calories: 55 Fat: 0.5g Carbohydrates: 14g Fiber: 3g Protein: 1g**

187. Melon Apple Cooler

Difficulty: Easy **Preparation Time:** 12 minutes

Cooking Time: 0 minutes **Serving:** 2 servings

Ingredients:

- 1/2 ripe honeydew melon, peeled and chopped
- 1 green apple, cored and chopped
- 1/4 cup fresh mint leaves
- 1 lime, juiced
- 1/2 cup of cold water
- Ice cubes (optional)

Instructions:

1. Add the chopped honeydew melon, green apple, and fresh mint leaves to a blender.
2. Blend the ingredients at a high speed until they are well mixed.
3. Pour the mixture into a large bowl through a fine mesh strainer to remove any solids.
4. Add the lime juice and cold water to the mixture and stir well.
5. If desired, add ice cubes to the mixture to make it cold and refreshing.
6. Pour the drink into glasses and serve.

Nutritional Values per Person: Calories: 63 Fat: 0.2g Carbohydrates: 16g Fiber: 2.1g Protein: 0.9g

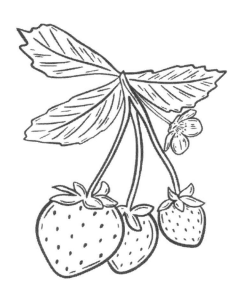

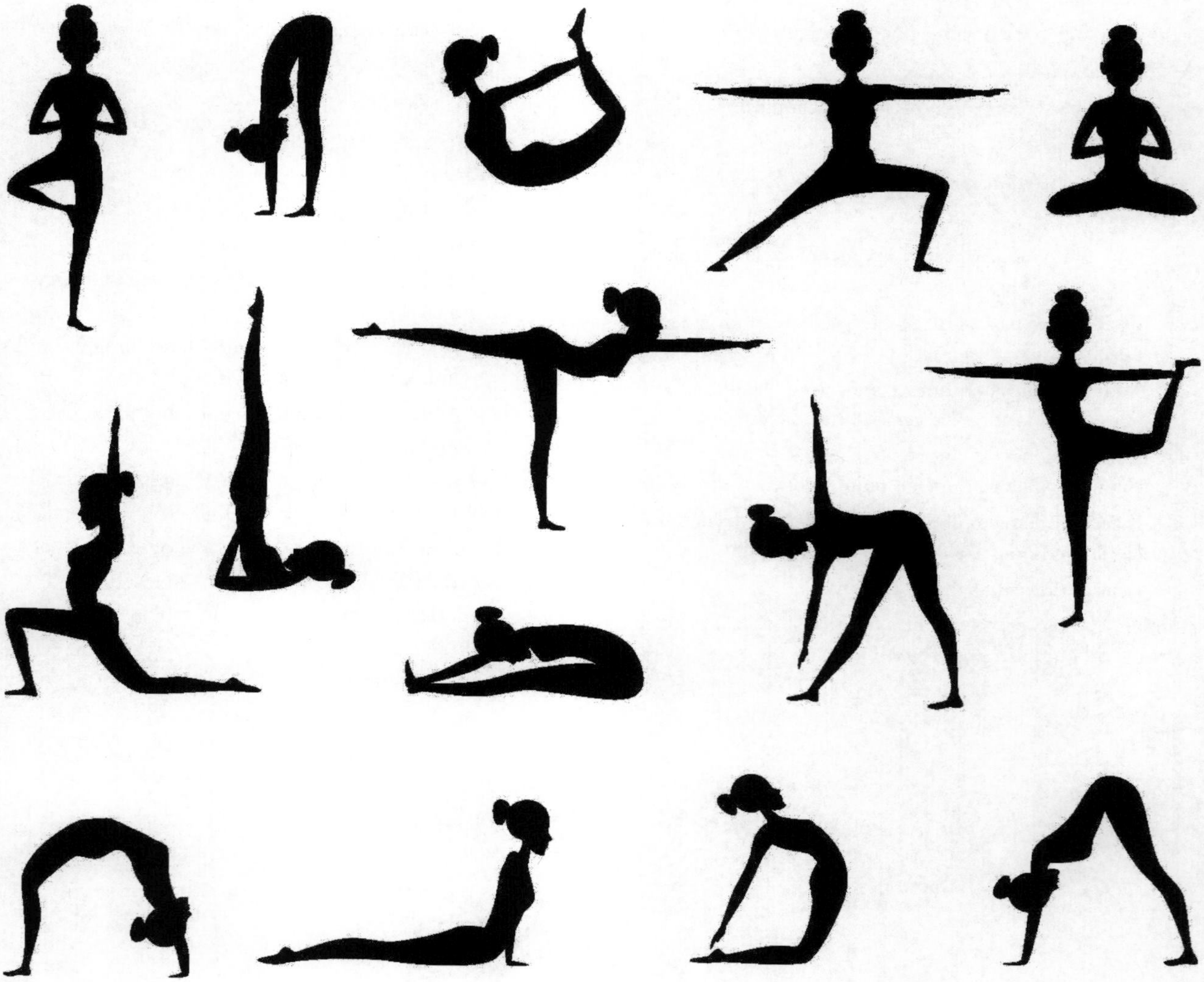

Recommended Physical Exercises

These physical exercises are ideal for people who suffer from fatty liver disease and can be performed in the comfort of their own home without any specialized equipment. Physical activity is known to play a critical role in improving liver health, reducing inflammation, and aiding in weight loss. The exercises listed here are low-impact and easy to perform, making them perfect for people with limited mobility or who are new to exercise. It's always important to consult your doctor before starting any exercise regimen to ensure it's safe for you. So, start incorporating these exercises into your daily routine and take a step towards a healthier liver and improved overall wellbeing.

1. Walking: Walking for 30 minutes or more every day.
2. Mountain Pose Standing: Keep the back straight and arms at the sides of the body. Inhale deeply and raise the arms above the head, then exhale as you lower the arms to the sides. Repeat for 5-10 breaths.
3. Chair Squat: Stand in front of a sturdy chair with feet shoulder-width apart. Keep your back straight, bend your knees, and lower yourself towards the chair. Stop when your glutes touch the seat and then rise up again. Do this for 10-15 repetitions.
4. Knee to Chest Stretch: Lie on your back with your knees bent and feet flat on the ground. Bring one knee to your chest and hold it with both hands. Hold for 10-15 seconds before moving to the other leg. Do this stretch 3-5 times on each leg.
5. Plank: Start in a push-up position with straight arms and hands shoulder-width apart. Keep the body straight from head to toes for 10-15 seconds. Repeat for 5-10 repetitions.
6. Leg Extension: Sit on a chair with a straight back and feet flat on the ground. Hold the armrests and extend one leg in front of you. Hold for 5-10 seconds before lowering it again. Repeat this for 10 repetitions on each leg.
7. Wall Push-Ups: Stand facing a wall with feet shoulder-width apart. Place hands on the wall at shoulder height and slightly wider than the shoulders. Lower the body towards the wall by bending the arms. Push back to the starting position. Do this for 10-15 repetitions.
8. Bridge: Lie on your back with your knees bent and feet flat on the ground. Raise your hips towards the ceiling while keeping the shoulders and feet on the ground. Hold for 5-10 seconds before lowering the hips again. Do this for 10-15 repetitions.
9. Seated Abdominal Twist: Sit on a chair with a straight back and feet flat on the ground. Clasp the hands in front of you and twist the torso to the right. Hold for 5-10 seconds before twisting to the left. Do this for 10-15 repetitions on each side.
10. Standing Toe Touch: Stand with feet shoulder-width apart. Lean forward and touch your toes while keeping the legs straight. Hold for 10-15 seconds before rising up again. Do this for 10-15 repetitions

Remember to always consult your doctor before starting any exercise program, especially if you have health problems.

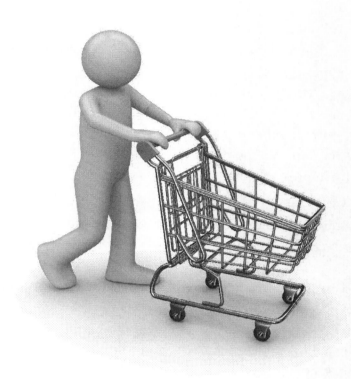

Shopping List

Produce:

- Sweet potatoes

- Avocado

- Eggs

- Mushrooms

- Spinach

- Tomatoes

- Berries (strawberries, blueberries, raspberries, etc.)

- Bananas

- Lemons

- Limes

- Garlic

- Onions

- Cucumbers

- Carrots

- Bell peppers (red, yellow, green)

- Broccoli

- Cauliflower

- Beets

- Radishes

- Zucchini

- Squash

- Green beans

- Salad greens (lettuce, spinach, arugula, etc.)

- Cilantro

- Basil

- Mint

- Ginger

- Apples

- Grapefruit

Pantry:

- Quinoa

- Rolled oats

- Almond flour

- Walnuts

- Almonds

- Chia seeds

- Peanut butter

- Canned chickpeas

- Canned mixed beans

- Lentils

- Brown rice

- Whole wheat pasta

- Farro

- Barley

- Millet

- Wheat berries

- Canned diced tomatoes

- Olive oil

- Balsamic vinegar

- Apple cider vinegar

- Coconut flour

- Ground cinnamon

- Honey

- Brown sugar

- Dark chocolate chips

- Soy sauce

- Sriracha sauce

- Dijon mustard

Meat, Fish and Seafood:

- Chicken breasts

- Turkey breast

- Turkey sausage

- Ground turkey

- Lamb chops

- Ground lamb

- Beef flank

- Salmon fillets

- Smoked salmon

- Halibut fillets

- Swordfish steaks

- Tuna steaks

- Shrimp

- Scallops

- Cod fillets

- Barramundi fillets

Dairy:

- Cottage cheese

- Greek yogurt

- Feta cheese

- Goat cheese

- Mozzarella cheese

Frozen:

- Mixed berries

- Mixed vegetables

Bakery:

- Bagels

- Whole wheat bread

Spices:

- Paprika

- Cumin

- Turmeric

- Chili powder

- Oregano

- Thyme

- Rosemary

- Ground coriander

- Black pepper

- Sea salt

- Green tea bags

- Coconut milk

Beverages:

- Unsweetened almond milk

Sweeteners:

- Stevia

Conclusion

In conclusion, the Fatty Liver Cookbook is an excellent resource for people looking to improve their liver health through diet. This cookbook not only offers delicious recipes but also provides essential information on fatty liver disease, its causes, and how certain foods can impact liver function. The recipes contained within the cookbook are easy to follow and use simple, wholesome ingredients. They are designed to be flavorful, satisfying, and help support liver function. The Fatty Liver Cookbook offers a clear and concise guide to eating for liver health, making it an essential resource for anyone looking to improve their wellbeing. Whether you're looking to manage fatty liver disease or just eat more healthily, this cookbook is a must-have in your kitchen.

28-Day Meal Plan

DAY	BREAKFAST	LUNCH	SNACKS	DINNER	DESSERTS
1	Quinoa Breakfast Bowl	Greek Salad	Roasted Chickpeas	Grilled Chicken with Vegetables	Fruit Salad
2	Low-Carb Scrambled Eggs	Beet and Goat Cheese Salad	Avocado and Cottage Cheese Toast	Pan-Seared Salmon with Sautéed Spinach	Chocolate Banana Smoothie
3	Sweet Potato Hash with Sausage and Eggs	Tuna Salad	Lemon and Ginger Cookies	Grilled Tuna Steaks with Lemon and Garlic	Apple Crisp
4	Cottage Cheese and Peach Salad	Egg Salad	Healthy Omega-3 Bagel	Chickpea Salad with Radishes and Carrots	Blueberry and Almond Flour Muffins
5	Green Smoothie Bowl	Grilled Shrimp Salad	Broccoli Bites	Grilled Lamb with Vegetables	Berry Sorbet
6	Omelette with Spinach and Mushrooms	Caprese Salad	Mexican Stuffed Bell Peppers	Baked Salmon with Asparagus	Chocolate ChiaPudding
7	Quinoa Porridge with Dried Fruit	Chicken Caesar Salad	Broiled Grapefruit with Honey and Cinnamon	Turkey Meatballs with Zucchini Noodles	Banana Oat Cookies
8	Coconut Flour Pancakes	Waldorf Salad	Hummus with Carrots and Cucumber	Turkey Chili with Sweet Potatoe	Tutti-Frutti Smoothie
9	Sweet Potato Toast with Avocado and Egg	Spinach Stuffed Mushrooms	Roasted Beet and Goat Cheese Salad	Grilled Chicken Kebabs with Vegetables	Fruit Salad
10	Tuna and Vegetable Frittata	Quinoa Salad	Crunchy Mozzarella Cauliflower	Seared Tuna Salad with Avocado	Apple Crisp
11	Dreamy Vanilla Chia Seed Pudding	Brown Basmati Rice Salad with Peppers and Almonds	Mediterranean Hummus Dip with Veggies	Grilled Turkey Cutlets	Chocolate Banana Smoothie
12	Mixed Berry Smoothie	Fatty Liver Fighting Salad	Baked Sweet Potato Chips	Chicken and Broccoli Air-Fry	Blueberry and Almond Flour Muffins
13	Avocado Toast with Smoked Salmon	Chicken Caesar Salad	Hummus with Carrots and Cucumber	Grilled Tuna Kebabs with Vegetables	Chocolate Chia Pudding
14	Coconut Quinoa Porridge with Fruit and Nuts	Spinach Salad	Broccoli Bites	Grilled Lamb Burger with Tzatziki Sauce	Fruit Salad
15	Smoothie with Beetroot and Carrot	Tuna Salad	Roasted Chickpeas	Grilled Lemon and Garlic Chicken Breasts	Banana Oat Cookies

16	Breakfast or Snack Option	Beet and Goat Cheese Salad	Mexican Stuffed Bell Peppers	Grilled Swordfish Steaks with Mint Pesto	Chocolate Banana Smoothie
17	Mixed Berry Smoothie	Quinoa Salad	Broiled Grapefruit with Honey and Cinnamon	Grilled Turkey Burger with Avocado and Tomato	Blueberry and Almond Flour Muffins
18	Sugar-free Oat and Banana Bars	Greek Salad	Crunchy Mozzarella Cauliflower	Grilled Chicken with Vegetables	Fruit Salad
19	Spinach and Bacon Frittata	Egg Salad	Mediterranean Hummus Dip with Veggies	Seared Scallops with Spinach Salad	Chocolate Chia Pudding
20	Low-Carb Blueberry Muffins	Fatty Liver Fighting Salad	Baked Sweet Potato Chips	Lamb Stew with Sweet Potato	Berry Sorbet
21	Quinoa Breakfast Bowl	Tuna Salad	Hummus with Carrots and Cucumber	Grilled Mahi-Mahi Sandwich with Avocado and Tomato	Apple Crisp
22	Matcha Tea Smoothie Bowl	Waldorf Salad	Roasted Chickpeas	Turkey Meatballs with Zucchini Noodles	Chocolate Banana Smoothie
23	Sweet Potato Pancakes	Caprese Salad	Mexican Stuffed Bell Peppers	Pan-Seared Barramundi with Lemon and Capers	Blueberry and Almond Flour Muffins
24	Chia Seed Pudding with Berries	Greek Salad	Broccoli Bites	Chicken Kofta	Fruit Salad
25	Low-Carb Scrambled Eggs	Grilled Shrimp Salad	Hummus with Carrots and Cucumber	Grilled Lemon and Herb Turkey Burger	Banana Oat Cookies
26	Quinoa Porridge with Dried Fruit	Spinach Salad	Crunchy Mozzarella Cauliflower	Grilled Halibut with Mango Salsa	Chocolate Chia Pudding
27	Coconut Flour Pancakes	Tuna Salad	Roasted Beet and Goat Cheese Salad	Grilled Lamb Chops with Mint Sauce	Berry Sorbet
28	Green Smoothie Bowl	Fatty Liver Fighting Salad	Baked Sweet Potato Chips	Grilled Rosemary Balsamic Chicken Skewers	Apple Crisp

Conversion Tables

Measure	Fluid OZ	TBSPP	Tsp	Liter & Milliliter
1 gallon	4 quarts	256 tbspp	768 tsp	3.75 l
4 cups	1 quart	64 tbspp	192 tsp	0,95 l
2 cups	1 pint	32 tbspp	96 tsp	470 ml
1 cup	8 oz	16 tbspp	48 tsp	237 ml
¾ cup	6 oz	12 tbspp	36 tsp	177 ml
2/3 cup	5 oz	11 tbspp	32 tsp	158 ml
½ cup	4 oz	8 tbspp	24 tsp	118 ml
1/3 cup	3 oz	5 tbspp	16 tsp	79 ml
¼ cup	2 oz	4 tbspp	12 tsp	59 ml
1/8 cup	1 oz	2 tbspp	6 tsp	30 ml
1/16 cup	0.5 oz	1 tbspp	3 tsp	15 ml

INDEX

Berry Blast Juice, 86

Berry Sorbet, 81

Blueberry and Almond Flour Muffins, 82

Breakfast Burrito, 18

Broccoli Bites, 25

Broiled Grapefruit with Honey and Cinnamon, 26

Broiled Scallops with Lemon Butter Sauce, 66

Brown Basmati Rice and Lentil Soup, 33

Brown Basmati Rice Salad with Peppers and Almonds, 31

Brown Basmati Rice with Squash and Walnuts, 32

Brown Rice and Lentil Bowl, 37

Brown Rice Pilaf with Spinach, 30

Caprese Salad, 76

Carrot and Ginger Juice, 84

Carrot and Pineapple Juice, 86

Chia Seed Pudding with Berries, 14

Chicken and Broccoli Air-Fry, 42

Chicken and Lentil Stew, 46

Chicken Caesar Salad, 76

Chicken Kofta, 57

Chickpea Hummus, 30

Chickpea Salad with Radishes and Carrots, 29

Chinese BBQ Chicken Wings, 54

Chinese Five Spice Chicken, 55

Chocolate Banana Smoothie, 80

Chocolate Chia Pudding, 82

Cilantro Lime Salmon, 59

Citrus Burst Juice, 85

Citrus Ginger Morning Juice, 86

Coconut Curry Fish Soup, 71

Coconut Flour Pancakes, 9

Coconut Quinoa Porridge with Fruit and Nuts, 18

Cottage Cheese and Peach Salad, 12

Cozy Apple Cinnamon Oatmeal, 12

Crunchy Mozzarella Cauliflower, 24

Dreamy Vanilla Chia Seed Pudding, 10

Egg Salad, 77

Farro Salad with Roasted Vegetables, 36

Fatty Liver Fighting Salad, 78

Fruit Salad, 80

Garlic Butter Shrimp Linguine, 66

Ginger Lemon Chicken Meatballs, 52

Greek Salad, 75

Greek Yogurt and Berries, 22

Greek Yogurt Chicken Salad, 54

Greek Yogurt Parfait, 15

Green Apple and Cucumber Juice, 85

Green Curry Chicken, 55

Green Curry Fish, 72

Green Detox Juice, 84

Green Smoothie Bowl, 11

Green Yogurt and Mixed Berries Bowl, 81

Grilled Chicken Breasts with Mango Salsa, 48

Grilled Chicken Kebabs with Vegetables, 47

Grilled Chicken with Roasted Beets, 44

Grilled Chicken with Vegetables, 41

Grilled Halibut with Mango Salsa, 64

Grilled Herb and Mustard Chicken Thighs, 50

Grilled Lamb Burger with Tzatziki Sauce, 49

Grilled Lamb Chops with Mint Sauce, 47

Grilled Lamb with Vegetables, 42

Grilled Lemon and Garlic Chicken Breasts, 49

Grilled Lemon and Herb Turkey Burger, 50

Grilled Mahi Mahi with Avocado and Tomato Salsa, 68

Grilled Mahi-Mahi Sandwich with Avocado and Tomato, 70

Grilled Rosemary Balsamic Chicken Skewers, 50

Grilled Shrimp Salad, 75

Grilled Shrimp Tacos with Avocado Salsa, 64

Grilled Swordfish Steaks with Mint Pesto, 67

Grilled Swordfish with Tomato Olive Relish, 68

Grilled Tuna Kebabs with Vegetables, 63

Grilled Tuna Steaks with Lemon and Garlic, 63

Grilled Turkey Burger with Avocado and Tomato, 48

Grilled Turkey Cutlets, 46

Grilled Turkey Skewers with Bell Peppers and Onions, 48

Gypsy Toast, 9

Healthy Omega-3 Bagel, 24

Healthy Pesto Pork Tenderloin Breakfast Bowl, 19

Healthy Smoked Salmon Breakfast Bagel, 11

Hearty Fish Soup, 73

Honey Mustard Chicken, 54

Hummus with Carrots and Cucumber, 24

Lamb Meatballs with Mint, 56

Lamb Stew with Sweet Potato, 46

Larb Gai (Thai Minced Chicken Salad), 57

Lemon and Ginger Cookies, 26

Lemon Herb Grilled Shrimp Skewers, 66

Lemon-Dill Grilled Salmon, 60

Low-Carb Blueberry Muffins, 16

Low-carb Scrambled Eggs, 8

Matcha Tea Smoothie Bowl, 20

Mediterranean Herb Lamb Meatballs, 51

Mediterranean Herb-Roasted Turkey Breast, 53

Mediterranean Hummus Dip with Veggies, 23

Melon Apple Cooler, 87

Mexican Stuffed Bell Peppers, 25

Millet and Chickpea Bowl, 38

Mixed Bean and Vegetable Soup, 30

Mixed Berry Smoothie, 14

Mixed Vegetable Lentil Soup, 29

Oatmeal Raisin Cookies, 26

Omelette with Spinach and Mushrooms, 11

Pan-Seared Barramundi with Lemon and Capers, 68

Pan-Seared Salmon with Sautéed Spinach, 59

Peanut Butter and Banana Cookies, 27

Peanut Butter Banana Smoothie, 14

Pineapple and Kale Juice, 84

Poached Cod with Lemon Butter Sauce, 67

Poached Salmon with Herbs, 61

Quinoa and Veggie Stuffed Peppers, 37

Quinoa Breakfast Bowl, 8

Quinoa Porridge with Dried Fruit, 15

Quinoa Salad, 78

Roasted Beet and Goat Cheese Salad, 25

Roasted Chickpeas, 23

Salmon Air-Fry, 60

Salmon Burger with Avocado Sauce, 69

Salmon Cakes, 59

Salt Cod in Tomato Sauce, 62

Salt Cod with Fennel and Tomatoes, 61

Scrambled Eggs with Tomatoes and Spinach, 15

Seafood Stew with Tomatoes and Garlic, 67

Seared Scallops with Spinach Salad, 69

Seared Tuna Salad with Avocado, 63

Smoothie with Beetroot and Carrot, 13

Spinach and Bacon Frittata, 17

Spinach and Mushroom Omelet, 13

Spinach Salad, 77

Spinach Stuffed Mushrooms, 23

Steamed Cod with Vegetables in Lemon Broth, 64

Steamed Fish with Ginger and Scallions, 71

Sugar-free Oat and Banana Bars, 19

Sweet Potato Hash with Sausage and Eggs, 10

Sweet Potato Pancakes, 20

Sweet Potato Toast with Avocado and Egg, 10

Tangy Green Juice, 87

Thai Basil Chicken, 55

Tom Kha Gai (Coconut Milk Soup with Chicken), 56

Tom Yum Soup with Fish, 72

Tuna and Vegetable Frittata, 12

Tuna Burger with Cucumber Yogurt Sauce, 69

Tuna Salad, 76

Tuna Salad and Cucumber Slices, 22

Tuna Salad Sandwich with Greek Yogurt and Celery, 70

Turkey and Butternut Squash Stew, 47

Turkey and Spinach Burger, 45

Turkey and Sugar Snap Pea Meatballs, 53

Turkey and Sweet Potato Burger, 45

Turkey and Vegetables Chili, 43

Turkey Chili with Sweet Potatoes, 44

Turkey Fajitas with Peppers and Onions, 52

Turkey Meatballs, 41

Turkey Meatballs with Zucchini Noodles, 43

Turkey Zucchini Meatballs, 51

Turmeric and Orange Juice, 85

Tutti-Frutti Smoothie, 80

Veggie and Cheese Omelet, 16

Waldorf Salad, 77

Watermelon and Mint Juice, 85

Wheat Berry and Broccoli Salad, 39

Whole Wheat Fettuccine with Shrimp and Tomato Sauce, 35

Whole Wheat Linguine with Lemon and Garlic Sauce, 34

Whole Wheat Pasta with Tuna and Tomato Sauce, 34

Whole Wheat Penne with Chicken and Broccoli, 36

Whole Wheat Spaghetti with Broccoli Sauce, 33

Whole Wheat Spaghetti with Spinach and Mushroom Sauce, 35

Wild Rice and Mushroom Pilaf, 32

Wild Rice Salad with Broccoli, 31

Thank you for making it this far. I have worked hard on this book, I hope you enjoyed it. A positive review on Amazon would help me a lot. Roslin Shelton.

Made in the USA
Middletown, DE
13 October 2023

40754906R00066